"Achieve Your Ultimate ...., *Natural, and Mind-Body Medicine"*

Whole Pharmacy

Reversing the Trends of Disease in an Over-Medicated Society

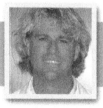

Robert Kress, RPh
The Whole Pharmacist

Hidden truths, alternatives
and complements to the
"modern day diseases" that
are destroying your health
and stealing your wealth

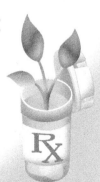

"Achieve Your Ultimate Health through Lifestyle, Natural, and Mind-Body Medicine"

Whole Pharmacy

Reversing the Trends of Disease in an Over-Medicated Society

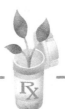

*"Liberty is to the collective body, what
health is to every individual body.
Without health no pleasure can be
tasted by man; without liberty, no
happiness can be enjoyed by society."*

-Thomas Jefferson

"This book is dedicated to all who have realized that ultimate wellbeing exists in the responsibility we take in our own
health, and the freedom that it provides us.

Thanks to all of the integrative researchers and practitioners who have
led the way, and those who continue to carry the torch
of righting the direction of the health of our society.

To my wife Amy for whom without, this book never would have been
written, this journey I would never have taking. I look forward to
continuing our journey for years ahead."

Table of Contents

Forward

> "*I always thought of myself as a humanities person as a kid, but I liked electronics. Then I read something that one of my heroes, Edwin Land of Polaroid, said about the importance of people who could stand at the intersection of humanities and sciences, and I decided that's what I wanted to do.*"

- Steve Jobs

In his biography of Steve Jobs, author, Walter Isaacson then went on to say,

> "*The creativity that can occur when a feel for both the humanities and the sciences combine in one strong personality was a topic that most interested me in my biographies of both Ben Franklin and Albert Einstein, and I believe it will be a key to creating innovative economies in the 21'st Century.*"

I believe that in medicine we can choose to reside at the intersection of humanities and science, and there is a bright future ahead for the health, wellness and wealth of our society- but simple shifts in perception and action leading to major change must occur.

Our dominant western medical system itself has grown to reside at the intersection of lack of morals and sciences, and has gotten there on the backs of greed, manipulation, and strong arm tactics.

We must decide which intersection to step off from, and which road to travel. Utilizing the great advances of modern day sciences combined with age old traditions of healing, for the benefit of our nation's health and economies. This will require recognizing the reality where the medical system is now, how it got here, and demanding a change from ourselves, patients, health care practitioners, industries and policymakers.

Robert Kress, RPH - The Whole Pharmacist

Introduction

Don't get me wrong... I am not totally against medications, just mostly. There are instances where medications have their place, certainly in cases of emergency, lives have been saved and incredible advancements made. Although the mass over usage of medications, I believe is unnecessary, and replaceable by lifestyle, diet, and natural medicine such as vitamins and herbs.

What is it that I don't like about prescription medications, especially being a pharmacist, you ask? 6 things!

1) Side-effects they can cause

2) Interactions with other medications and supplements

3) They often acidify the body, throwing off the healthy alkaline balance, open up the body to disease

4) They lead to nutrient depletions

5) They only mask symptoms, they do not get to the root of the problem

6) Financially unsustainable

Optimal healing is about balance-. *Dis-ease* is about imbalance. For the most part a prescription medication will only cover up the symptoms, or silence the cry from within for balance.

Every day I hear from clients who are sick and tired of feeling sick and tired, or they forget what it feels like to feel good. They are sick and tired of the 'magic bullet' of drugs not working, and feeling they are only treading water and not getting better, frustrated with lack of time and options from their practitioners.

Practitioners are the same, they are realizing that we are in an over-medicated society; they are frustrated with their choices and many are looking for alternatives to help their patients. Of course we will always have our pill pushing prescribers, pill vendor pharmacists, and patients who are just fine with numbing themselves from reality; but there is a very big transition of people wanting more for their life and from their health.

Over 70% of Americans are on prescription drugs and as a nation we keep getting sicker- do you see the relationship here? If you were to ask me what is the main problem with the health care system? Why does the United States spend the most money, and have the worst health of other industrialized nations, despite that 75% of all health care expenditures are spent on preventable diseases? My answer is simple- it's the system itself.

Our health has been bought and sold many times over, providing benefits for the multinational food, pharmaceutical and insurance industries, while the citizens foot the bill, costing them their wealth as well as their health.

Our health care system is not about caring for and promoting health, our health care system is a disease management system, keeping people just sick enough to be repeat customers. What we need to focus on and navigate towards is a system which is based around health promotion and disease prevention- we need to find balance!

We need to shift focus, take responsibility back into our own hands and not hand our health over to this system which generates a tremendous amount of revenue for a few industries (i.e. - pharmaceutical, medical devices, insurers), and leaves the masses with higher premiums and increasing rates of disease.

My intention in writing this book is to offer readers a complete perspective on health, help clear the confusion of what they hear on TV, one that serves as a guide to help navigate through what I consider to be an over-medicated society and an over-medication driven health care system.

I am not saying that Pharma has no place; I am just saying they are taking up too much space. Being a conventional pharmacist as well as a practitioner of many alternative and holistic practices of health, is what makes this view on the situation unique.

There is a paradigm shift at hand in regards to the health of our society. A fork in the road has appeared and it is up to us as individuals to decide which path to travel; a path of self-responsibility and empowered health, or one of the maintenance of disease. Living the path of self-responsibility and empowered health is all about living from a true choice in the present moment rather than being run by society's programming, conditioning from your past, and ultimately being controlled by ego.

Albert Einstein claimed that, *"the problems of the world would not be solved at the same level of thinking we were at when we created them."* I believe this is exactly the case with our current medical system and the climate that exists in health care. A different level of thinking requires a different perception and view of the world and oneself, and that often requires taking different actions. The overprescribing of medications in our society is a real problem, and one's prescription needs are only a symptom of the challenges in our modern day world, the direction our medical system has evolved, and the choices patients make. This is a pattern that plays upon the weakness of one's ego, and is perpetuated through fear.

I will be sharing with you some truths which might have been misguiding you or a loved one, the benefit of taking responsibility for your own health, and seeking out the most qualified health care practitioners to help you on your path while seeing them as partners and advisors to your health, instead of the end all experts.

Most of this information you most likely will not hear at your next doctors visit or trip to the pharmacy (I would be psyched if you did- and we are seeing a growing number of all practitioners in this direction), although it is exactly what you need to know about living a healthy life in a system of medical care that offers a misguided and biased focus.

These are the lessons I share with my customers and clients on a regular basis and picked up in my years as a pharmacist and a nutritionist seeking other solutions for people's problems of health- away from an over-medicated society.

My wife and I have studied many different areas of health and wellness; conventional pharmacy and medicine, Reiki, Auricular acupuncture, EFT (emotional freedom technique). I have received my certification in clinical nutrition, completed advanced studies in the art of pharmaceutical compounding, and have dived head first into areas of mind-body medicine, meditation, homeopathy and other disciplines which are often not on the standard of care menu in your local pharmacy- all in my quest to find a better way of health care.

I have spent many years coaching other pharmacists on how to bring natural medicine into their practice. I have created C.E.'s (continuing education) to train pharmacists, staff and nurses in complementary therapies through nutrition and holistic medicine, and now I want to bring this all to you. In this book we will be addressing some of the hidden truths behind our system of medicine which lead people down the wrong path, although this book is not about pointing fingers. This book is about empowerment, so we will also be sharing with you the simple truths and tips for radical change in your health, regardless of where your state of health exists today.

This book is divided into four sections. First, I will be addressing the state of our society's health today, and how we got here by being driven by the health care system itself. Next, I will address the major areas in which I feel peoples' health have been hijacked, and offer you alternatives and complements. Section three is about the healing path, and it contains some of my favorite tools, tips, and resources to healing, which then flows into section four offering a suggestion of daily health minded and physical actions- what I like to call, "The Whole Health Prescription of Simple Steps for Radical Changes to Your Health."

Health matters. Health is about personal growth as much as relationships, wealth, and happiness. When you think about it, pretty much everything bad that life can throw at you, such as business, or relationships, or politics will not kill you...not so with health.

Your health is the sum of every element of your life. Every element in your life has the ability to affect your health; from your finances, to your relationships, to your thoughts, - everything. This is why I believe looking at ones health in a holistic manner, regardless of where one is today, is the most important thing you can do for yourself.

In some cases, someone might think it will take nothing less than a miracle to get them well, this is a defeating belief. I believe miracles in health can happen, although I want you to understand what I mean by this. I am not saying it's magic; we are not pulling a rabbit out of a hat. You will see some references in this book alluding to the book, "*A Course in Miracles*", and when I read this book I had a major ah ha moment. First, one must understand that the authors were themselves involved in the conventional medical paradigm, as clinical psychologists at Columbia University.

The book was the result of a simple shift in their perception- that's exactly what a miracle is as they describe it. Miracles are simple shifts in one's perception which lead to the behavioral follow up aligned with our true desires, and then we get results. While simple, this doesn't mean we should treat these simple shifts lightly. As is outlined in the course, "*Miracles transcend the body. They are sudden shifts into invisibility, away from the bodily level. That is why they heal.*"

Me and Pharmacy

I might not be considered as your "average" pharmacist, but fortunately there are growing numbers of pharmacists and other practitioners opening up to the practice of integrative medicine.

Ever since I got my pharmacy license it seemed as if I was trying to get out of the profession of pharmacy. Even when I was in pharmacy school I knew that something was wrong. At that time we were seeing the increases in prescription psychotropic drugs such as Prozac, and even family pets were being put on such drugs- it was a new kind of insanity.

It was 1995 and I made a pact with myself that I would be out of the practice of pharmacy by the year 2000. I have broken that pact with myself, and am happy I did. At the time I was disenchanted with the practice of pharmacy, feeling like a pill mill and watching people go on the merry-go-round of prescription therapy, treating drug side-effects with more drugs, it was madness and in many cases it's still the same today.

So, we ran away. In the summer of 1995, my wife and I made our exodus from the Philadelphia area and headed west with all of our worldly possessions and our chocolate lab, Hannah, in tow. After a 3 month road trip we ended up in Jackson Hole Wyoming where for the next 8 plus years I ran a retail pharmacy in a quintessential ski town…kind of a dream come true. The weird thing is that I daydreamed about this. It wasn't Jackson Hole, heck I never even knew there were mountains in Wyoming, - I thought Colorado was going to be my dream come true.

I actually daydreamed about working in a ski town and being able to leave work and be on the mountain in a matter of minutes- this became my reality. It turns out that Jackson Hole was the place which I needed to experience certain influence's to take my career to the next level. This is just one example we will be addressing later on showing how one's reality can change when guided by simple shifts in perception, on what one focuses on and emotionalizes.

After eight and one-half years in Jackson, we knew it was time to move on, and this change made me realize that pharmacy was my place to be, albeit, not the kind of pharmacy the prescription driven medical system had in mind.

During our time in Jackson Hole, I was introduced to the power of mind-body medicine; I came across it in my own 'crisis of health,' where I ended up on the operating table for back surgery. What I quickly learned after the surgery was that while I was 'healed', that the pain could still come back in the absence of any physical stressors, although there was a strong connection to mental and emotional stressors. I also learned that by doing something physical (snowboarding only about a month after surgery) it did not produce the pain as long as I was doing something which brought positive emotions such as pleasure, creativity and fun.

I then caught on to the growing industry of pharmacy compounding and realized I could create my own pharmacy based on compounding and nutrition while not carrying any "regular prescription or OTC drugs" on my shelves- thus I created what was my definition of the perfect pharmacy.

My experience with compounding led me to accreditation as a CCN (certified clinical nutritionist) via the Clinical Nutrition Certification Board (CNCB). Our pharmacy soon grew into a wellness clinic which housed a pharmacy along with other integrative practitioners such as doctors, nutritionists, skin care specialists and massage therapists.

Today I work with other like-minded health care practitioners, ones who are looking to expand into nutrition and other complementary services. As you will see, I have great hope for the direction that medicine is going and have a sound reason for doing so. I believe that as a culture if we focus on taking back responsibility and step toward the empowerment of health, that we will find the answer to limitless health and sustainable, affordable medicine..

Why I Have Written This Book

When asked what surprised him most about humanity, The Dali Lama responded;

> *"Man. Because he sacrifices his health in order to make money. Then he sacrifices money to recuperate his health. And then he is so anxious about the future that he does not enjoy the present; the result being that he does not live in the present or the future; he lives as if he is never going to die, and then dies having never really lived."*

This response by the Dali Lama is the reality of where much of our society is at. I know this is not what most people want, and I also feel people get so caught up in the cycle that the result of "having never really lived" is inevitable. This is why I have written this book.

I feel it's time has come. We sit at a very unique juncture in history; I like to think we on the verge of a healthy renaissance, I think more and more people are recognizing this and are more willing to make a change than ever before- some out of preventative choice, others out of necessity. This book has been rolling around in my brain for a very long time. I feel today, worldwide, people are ready to make such changes of perceptions, actions and habits to reverse the paths many have gone towards ill health, for themselves and for their loved ones.

Over the past Century, our medical system has operated mainly around pharmaceutical care. Because of this, your neighborhood pharmacy often finds itself front and center of your health care experience. Where there have been many advancements under this model, it has become evident that a complementary approach is the best option to treat someone's health over the long haul.

A recent report (2013) found that the United States of America is unhealthier than 16 other developed countries. The report, which was compiled by the National Research Council and the Institutes of Medicine, found that, despite the fact that Americans spend the most money per year on healthcare, we're not healthier or living longer than other countries.

Of the health areas studied, Americans ranked worse than other countries in nine categories, including, among others, drug abuse, heart disease, obesity and diabetes, and lung disease- all very preventable. The study found that U.S. men live the shortest lives of all 16 countries at 76 years, and U.S. women ranked second-to-last at just less than 81 years. Americans are more likely to die younger because of illnesses like obesity and heart disease.

In a large national survey in 2012, it was found that only 13 percent of baby boomers, reported being in "excellent" health in middle age. This is compared to 32 percent of the previous generation who said the same at the same stage of life- this is a major difference and a trend we do not want to continue.

Fortunately there is a rising consciousness based on the truth about the foods that we eat, and transparency is becoming front and center about how our health has been hijacked. The pharmaceutical industries approval rating is similar to Wall Street banks, as they have continually shown examples of how they have lost their purpose, their morals- all the while people want to get healthier and are taking action and taking back responsibility.

This book fills a unique spot, and provides the tools and information to help others empower themselves to have ultimate health in an over-medicated society and where there is a medical system that is failing us.

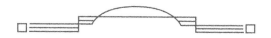

Part I:

TREADING WATER

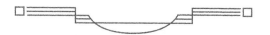

Chapter 1

A System That Needs Fixing

I will be using the term conventional medicine to refer to our current, allopathic, prescription and surgery based western medical system. I see many people call this traditional, although what I consider traditional is the holistic model I am about to share with you. I will be using the terms holistic and integrative to refer to a balanced system of health, one that recognizes all options of healing; from the mind, emotions, and body, utilizing the best options in regards to the patient. This might include nutrition, homeopathy, yoga, meditation and other modalities of healing.

Pharmageddon is upon us and the pharmaceutical drug cartel is stealing our nation's health, killing hundreds of people on a daily basis and bankrupting the citizens. This current conventional medical system is broken, and it has been broken for a very long time. There have been many great advances, and there are many morally sound practitioners whose goal is to fight disease, although as you will see through much greed and desire for control, the system at large needs a major over-haul and it starts with us.

A recent report has indicated that nearly 70% of Americans take at least 1 prescription drug daily, and over ½ take at least 2 prescriptions. According to the Centers for Disease Control and Prevention, approximately 76% of patients 60 years and older take at least 2 prescription drugs, and 37% take at least 5 prescription drugs. So as you can see, pharmaceutical therapy is the "norm," now let's take a look at some sobering facts which this "norm" has brought us:

- Adverse drug reactions cause injuries or death in 1 of 5 hospital patients.

- Every day over 290 people are killed by FDA approved prescription drugs, that's over 106,000 people each year.

- Expenditures on prescription drugs reached $250 billion in 2009, 12% of total health care spending.

- According to the groundbreaking 2003 medical report *Death by Medicine*, by Drs. Gary Null, Carolyn Dean, Martin Feldman, Debora Rasio and Dorothy Smith, 783,936 people in the United States die every year from conventional medicine mistakes. 106,000 due to drug side-effects, 98,000 due to medical errors, 88,000 due to infections, 32,000 due to surgery, and 37,000 due to unnecessary procedures.

- Fifty years ago, Americans spent approximately 16 percent of their disposable income on food and 5 percent on health care. In 2010, they spent 7 percent on food and 17 percent on health care.

And I ask you, why is no one in Washington is even talking about this? The FDA will impose regulations and fines, which essentially amount to little more than a slap on the wrist for major pharmaceutical companies, and this is done long after people have been injured and lives have been lost.

Instead you hear about regulations and mandates to give people more poison such as vaccination mandates, law makers looking for more control over the nutrition industry, while non-pasteurized milk products or even whole foods sellers are targeted and attacked with industry regulators brandishing firearms as if they are making a sting on an illegal drug operation. All the while, over ¾ of a million people are dying each year due to this conventional medical model- this is truly insanity. Finally, in what seems to be a major slap in the face to the public at large, the Supreme Court has recently ruled that drug companies are exempt from law suits- talk about being rewarded for bad behavior.

We are now a culture with two distinct systems of health, one that is about self-responsibility and empowerment of health, and another which is about the maintenance of disease and volunteered victimization by the participants.

Let me make this clear. I am not totally against conventional allopathic medicine, but it needs some serious fixing. I recognize that prescriptions and surgery are often needed to jump start our healing path, although people are still dying and not healing due to unnecessary surgeries and drug therapy.

We have a great system of emergency medicine; we have seen many times our modern-day system of health care provide wonderful healing from disease, although our medical system fails us after the emergency. As far as maintenance and preventative health, one must look to the natural and integrative side, providing alternative or complementary therapy to the allopathic model. We must expand into the mind-body; recognize that there is a work/life purpose to an empowering life, as well as healthy relationships, spirituality, and creativity.

I do not think most doctors, pharmacists and other health care practitioners are bad people or have evil intentions. For the most part, even the ones who may not agree with much of what I say have the best intentions for their patients' health. Although, they might act out of fear and ignorance, which serves no benefit to their patients.

In this book you are going to find that I am a realist, and I believe that it is realistic to have abundant, empowered health. I am not some hyped type A trainer hitting the gym at 5 am and saying that you have to as well to attain health, nor am I a person writing a book who has had a relatively un-stressful life, born with a silver spoon in their mouth fed to me by a personal chef, promising great results that often exist only to those who got lucky in the gene pool.

I understand what our society is going through, see the challenges, realize the problems and would like to shed light on the solutions. I understand anyone can improve on their current health path through a healthy balance of diet and lifestyle, and complimentary forms of therapy while avoiding the prescription merry-go-round.

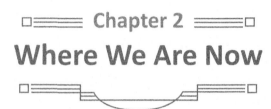

Chapter 2
Where We Are Now

"Over the past two decades the pharmaceutical industry has moved very far from its original high purpose of discovering and producing useful, new drugs. Now primarily a marketing machine to sell drugs of dubious benefit, the industry uses its wealth and power to corrupt every institution that might stand in its way, including the US Congress, the FDA, academic medical centers, and the medical profession itself."

- **Marcia Angell MD**, *Former editor of the New England Journal of Medicine*

I don't know if truer words have ever been spoken. Dr. Angell's first-hand experience from within the system, has undoubtedly shown her some hard to face truths about a health care system that has seriously gone astray.

So is the answer increasing government regulations and influence on how it's going to be paid for and who is going to make the decisions? Heck no, to get out of this mess, we have to dismantle or opt-out of what is really wrong, regroup what we know works, and move ahead from there.

Healthy living is not and should not be about politics, it's about values towards health and separation from the ego mind. While the folks in Washington are arguing who is going to pay for illness care and how to get their hands deeper into our wallets, should we not be focusing on how to create a healthier culture? What do you value and desire? A healthy and vibrant lifestyle, free of disease allowing you the freedom to do what you want? Or is it a system of lemming care, where you do not empower yourself, but instead rely on the judgment and actions of others to tell you how healthy, or sick you can and will be? I choose the former, and within this choice come self-responsibility, the first step to empowered health and the avoidance of what I consider the 5 most addictive drugs dispensed to us from our ego mind; fear, blame, self-pity, negative self-talk, and the identity of illness.

A Shift Towards Self-Care

> *Doctors don't heal, optimally a doctor's job is to facilitate the body's healing process by adding whatever is lacking when self-healing falters.* - Deepak Chopra

I remember an article in the Whole Earth Catalog, Millennial Edition from 1994. The article was titled, *From Industrial-Age Medicine To Information-Age Health Care,* and suffice to say, this article was way ahead of its time, and was already providing solutions for the growing problem in health care which has taken us to today, with the solution being a greater shift towards self-care.

The article highlighted both systems of medicine, where industrial age medicine encouraged professional care first (high dollar), regardless of the problem in health, and discourages self-care (low dollar). Information age health care is just the opposite where it encourages individual self-care first (low dollar) and discourages health care professionals (high dollar) as ultimate authorities, unless needed.

An interesting note is that the low dollar comes with more self-responsibility, and the high dollar is more akin to giving way one's responsibility. In the information age health care where many would agree we are needing to transition further to, there are 6 progressive steps which started at low dollar health care promoting self-responsibility and control and transitioned to high dollar medical treatment looking outsides one's self to health professionals if need be.

1. Individual Self-Care- Individual first attempts to prevent, recognize, manage and/or treat on their own.

2. Family and Friends- When individual self-care does not work or there are questions, people then turn to family, friends and neighbors for advice, information and support.

3. Self-help groups and networks- When the above groups are not sufficient, people turn to experienced self-helpers and support groups. The Internet has made this ever so more accessible and possible.

4. The Health Professional as Facilitator- Basic electronic communication between patients and professionals for the professional's expertise could cut costs, save time, and improve care. Professionals would put aside their authority role and serve as advisors, facilitators, and supporters of self-provided care. The assumption would be that even though professional consultation was needed, clients could successfully manage most aspects of most health problems on their own, which would provide a resolution of legal liability making health professionals more comfortable with this new role.

5. The Health Professional as Partner- Serious or chronic problems often require occasional or regular contact between professionals and patients whether it be phone, video, in office, home or hospital visits.

6. The Health Professional as Authority- This would involve emergency situations, as well as high tech interventions.

As you can see, this model puts responsibility in the patients' hands, although allows for needed intervention, support, consult from experts in the field. Every individual will approach this model from a different perspective, some needing one on one medical intervention expertise, others searching for the benefits of a medical professional in a "project manager" sort of way, while others, self-care will be their comfort zone.

If a transition towards self-responsibility was promoted and attained within our health care system this could dramatically cut health care expenses while improving health care outcomes. The only people I see not benefiting from this would be...you guessed it, the pharmaceutical cartel. One thing to understand is that the transition to information age medicine has made this possible, the internet brings with it its own challenges such as misinformation, hyped up and false marketing claims and more, thus the importance of aligning yourself with someone of expertise, in one way or another.

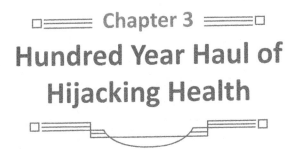

Chapter 3

Hundred Year Haul of Hijacking Health

I think it is important to understand just how our medical system has evolved in a relatively short amount of time. Within the hundred year haul of hijacking our health, a host of disease states have been added to the equation, relatively new to the existence of man and woman, although not so coincidentally in line with the advent of our conventional model of health.

Think about it, there are other systems of medicine, way older than our conventional, western model. Homeopathy is over 200 year's old, Traditional Chinese medicine and Ayurvedic medicine are both over 5000 years old with a great track record of success in regards to healing and safety, and all can be easily adapted in our 'western culture' way of life and medicine.

Here in the West, this system is very new, only about 100 years old. At the beginning of the 20Th century the medical landscape was a mixed bag of naturopaths, a growing industry of chemical based medicine, and of course your snake oil salesmen and charlatans.

At this time the medical landscape in America was ripe to be taken over, and the implementation of a takeover begun. In 1904 the American Medical Association (AMA) created what was known as The Council of Medical Education (CME) whose objective was to restructure the American medical educational system.

The CME appointed Abraham Flexner to conduct a survey to assess the American medical educational system. The results of this survey were released in 1910: known as the Flexner Report.

One could argue that mainstream medicine at the time was in the need of reform much the same way as our current industrial food complex and medical system is in need of overhaul; the end result supported the industrial side of medicine.

Abraham Flexner and the CME sought to eliminate a great number of medical schools as well as to limit the number of medical school graduates. They called for standardization of what medical schools taught and those not in accordance would have to merge or close their doors. Flexner recommended that medical schools appoint full-time clinical professors, who would basically fall under restrictions to how much income they could produce for themselves.

There were small proprietary schools of the day operating under a for-profit model. These schools stemmed from a tradition of folk-based medicine and allowed admittance of African Americans, women, and students of limited financial means. Proprietary schools did not fit into the Flexner formula and were recommended to close, leading to a profession predominately run by the white male elite.

Flexner clearly did not favor any form of medicine which did not advocate the use of treatments such as vaccinations and the rising chemical based patented medicine. Disciplines such as naturopathy and homeopathy opposed this agenda; the schools, which taught these disciplines, were told either to eliminate the courses from their curriculum or they would be forced to close their doors.

The impact of the Flexner report re-sculpted the practice of medicine in America. There became limited options of treatment and care; only chemical based patented medicine was taught and widely practiced, restraining and eliminating the disciplines of natural origin. This led to shortages of practitioners, less availability of care and increased costs (sound familiar?). Many gifted individuals of medicine were unable to obtain a degree due to lack of financial backing, and the pool of teachers became limited to narrow focused professors, many of whom lacked any aspiration to think beyond the standards set in place.

…If this sounds eerily familiar to what is happening today, it is. And as they say, "coincidences take a lot of planning."

This increasing control and bureaucracy has proven in the past and will most likely prove in the future to be counterproductive to the benefits of a free market and the health of our nation.

"But we are living longer" you might say, "Is this not the result of the pharma based medical system?" No. You see, we owe this to the true genius and innovation of the engineers who found ways to deal with sanitation issues which was one of the main reasons for the leading killers of the day-infectious disease. Contrary to what many believe, most vaccines came after the targeted health problems were reduced or eradicated by the solutions of sanitation and cleaner living. Vaccinations by a large part are just another shell game by the pharmaceutical industry based on bad or no science, sold on the formula of fabricated problem-reaction-solution, when in truth, largely unnecessary, but more on this later.

The years went on, and our nation began to develop other issues of health that 'under-developed' countries were not experiencing; heart disease, cancer, diabetes, depression, autism, and dementia related disorders and of course, increasing deaths from medications, even when properly prescribed. Why? Because we were in the treat the symptom prescription culture which has gone out of control.

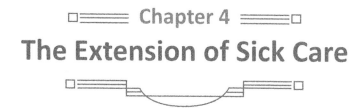

Chapter 4

The Extension of Sick Care

Standard of Care

There has been a medical standard of care which has been created which is essentially medical treatment guideline. Where in one aspect the intention might have been to provide guidelines for the safety and wellbeing of a patient, on the other hand it can act as a set of rules and dogma's that might actually prevent optimal care for a patient, due to practitioner's fear of "thinking outside the pill bottle" and stepping over the line.

For instance, standard of care can be perceived on a national level, local, or even within a medical system such as a hospital. As you will learn, saliva testing is the gold standard in the medical literature for assessment of hormones such as assessing adrenal stress with cortisol. I have seen firsthand large medical practices and hospital based systems not allow their practitioners to utilize these forms of testing calling it non-evidence based which is absolutely false. In such cases whether on regional, national, or even private levels, physicians can feel as if they are sticking their necks out, and can be subject to punishment if challenging this model of standard of care. In the end it's the patients who ultimately suffer.

Burying studies and Publication Bias

The conventional medical system often hides behind what is called evidence based medicine, which is basically approving drugs and treatments based off of scientific studies. So, if a drug is approved by the FDA, one would assume that every study done on this drug would be submitted to the FDA for review, as well as make it to peer review literature. Thus the FDA and active practitioners would have access to and be able to make its most informed decision if this drug really serves a unique purpose in treatment, that it is safe and effective, and appropriate for their patients.

You might be surprised to find out that this is often not the case.

Publication bias exists in all areas of medicine, and believe it or not ½ of all trials performed on drugs to be presented to the FDA for approval go missing in action and are not available to other practitioners or published in peer reviewed sources of literature. Studies get buried due to negative outcomes which if practitioners knew more about, would not bode well for the approval and prescribing of the drug. It is common practice that studies with positive findings are twice as likely to get published as studies with negative findings.

Dr. Ben Goldacre from Bad Pharma shared an example of such publication bias. Researchers focused on all anti-depressants which were approved over a 15 year period. All the trials that were submitted to the FDA for these 12 antidepressants which received FDA approval were studied. Of these studies there were 38 with positive results, and 36 with negative results. In peer reviewed journals where practitioners, patients and academics have access to make their own assessment, all but one of the positive resulting studies (37) were published, and only 3 of the negative resulting studies were published.

So, if you are a practitioner or academic doing your due diligence and researching a new drug, for the safety and effectiveness of your patients, or a patient doing their own research, in the case above you would have seen an overwhelming amount of studies for the positive, and few to the negative, most likely resulting in you prescribing this drug on full faith of safety and effectiveness. When in reality if you had the opportunity to look at all studies involved, you could come to the conclusion that bad vs. good is a draw and it might not be worth it to even try it based on safety and effectiveness.

As you can see, often times when your physician feels they are prescribing you a medication that can actually help, and be safe, their ability to make an objective decision is seriously hampered by buried studies not made available to them.

Let us take a look at just a few dangerous drugs approved by the FDA which will make you wonder if there was some form of publication bias due to the side-effects and issues that have come about after making it to market. You will probably recognize many of these from lawyer commercials on TV.

Vioxx

Vioxx, a blockbuster anti-inflammatory drug by Merck which was pulled off the market and the company agreed to pay $4.85 billion to settle nearly 27,000 lawsuits that claim the arthritis drug caused heart attacks and strokes. And as you will see, even with numerous studies presented to the FDA in support of such cardiac events, this still didn't stop the original FDA approval. Vioxx's danger first appeared in 1998 during a Merck study labeled 090. This study found nearly a seven-fold increase in heart attack risk with low dose Vioxx, which was ignored at its approval. In 2000, a Merck study named VIGOR found a five-fold increase in heart attack risk with high-dose Vioxx. Two years later, a large epidemiologic study reported a two-fold increase in heart attack risk with high-dose Vioxx. All the while the drug stayed on the market and doctors continued to prescribe Vioxx, which was sold in eighty countries, and reached $2.5 billion in sales in 2003. In 2004, FDA scientist David Graham estimated that Vioxx injured 88,000 to 139,000 Americans – 30 to 40% probably died.

Vioxx was not the only 'bad drug' in this class of anti-inflammatory medications known as cyclo-oxygenase-2 (COX 2) inhibitors which came to popularity due to a lower risk of developing ulcers as is the case with older drugs such as ibuprofen and naproxen. Bextra, another COX2 inhibitor from the drug company Searle was finally withdrawn from the U.S. market on April 7, 2005, due to its increased risk to lead to heart attacks and strokes. The thing is, before it was pulled, the FDA was warned by an FDA drug safety advisor, Dr. Furberg who insisted that his studies "Showed that Bextra is no different than Vioxx, and Pfizer is trying to suppress that information." Immediately thereafter, Dr. Furberg was barred by the FDA from serving on the panel responsible for considering the safety of COX 2 inhibitors. Knowing this information, are you comfortable to be taking other like medications such as Celebrex and Mobic whose packaging accompanies the warnings of increased chance of heart attacks and strokes?

Statin Drugs

Personally, I think this is a major case of "looking the other way" by the FDA. One of the darlings of the pharmaceutical industry over the last 20 years is a class of medications known as statins. While many Americans have developed a love affair with these drugs, very few are made aware of their negative side effects by their doctors or pharmacists- I see it every day. And the sad thing is, many pharmacists and physicians do not know (or believe when told) the scope of the problems statin drugs lead to. Cholesterol-lowering drugs can be silent killers. In a letter to the Archives of Internal Medicine, Uffe Ravnskov, M.D., Ph.D. and colleagues show that in two of the three clinical trials that included healthy people, the chance of survival was better without the use of cholesterol-lowering drugs.

Numerous medical journals have shown that cholesterol-lowering drugs significantly increase one's risk of suffering from deficiency of the energizing molecule CoEnzyme Q10 (CoQ10.) Low CoQ10 is associated with congestive heart failure, rhabdomyolysis (muscle deterioration causing pain and weakness), kidney failure, neurologic problems, increased risk of diabetes, breast cancer, problems with memory and loss of mental focus. CoQ10 is critical for mitochondrial and muscle health and finds its highest concentration in the heart, thus one might argue that we are adding insult to injury and that we are actually preventing healthy aging through statin therapy. Low CoQ10 levels are commonly found in people with heart disease.

Many times I have seen patients complain of muscle pain, and all the doctor does is put them on a different statin drug, all the while it has been proven that statins can damage muscle even in absence of elevated normal creatine kinase levels, which the usual indicator of muscle damage monitored with statin usage. Remember, a symptom is a call from within that there is a bigger problem brewing, and I don't think there could be a clearer example in drug therapy.

This coincides what has been reported in Europe, especially the U.K., where statin drugs have become a non-prescription favorite. The U.K. now has the dubious distinction of being the only country where statins can be purchased over-the-counter, and the amount of statin consumption there has increased more than 120% in recent years. Increasingly, orthopedic clinics are seeing patients whose problems turn out to be solvable by simply terminating statin therapy.

Zyprexa

Zyprexa is an antipsychotic medication, and yet another alarming example of FDA-approved drugs being unsafe with questionable effectiveness. It was reported in the New York Times that Eli Lilly worked to downplay the links between the drug and obesity, increased blood sugar levels and increased diabetes risk.

Clinical trials lasting a mere six weeks showed that the drug was linked to life-threatening side effects requiring hospitalization in 22% of those treated. A weight gain of 50-70 pounds was common among users. Studies showed that users were ten times more likely to suffer from Type-II diabetes as a result of taking the drug short term, and as many of you know, type II diabetes and weight gain go hand in hand.

During the six-week clinical trials for Zyprexa there were twenty deaths. Among these deaths, twelve were suicides. Dr. David Healy has stated that clinical trials surrounding Zyprexa "Demonstrate a higher death rate on Zyprexa than on any other antipsychotic ever recorded." I distinctly remember dispensing this medication when it came out, and not being made aware of any of this information that would have been useful for me and other practitioners in counseling our patients.

Tamiflu

Tamiflu, a drug made by Roche has been at the center of this study debate for years. Tamiflu which is FDA approved for treatment of the swine and seasonal flu comes with some strong and relevant questions in regards to its efficacy and safety. The trouble is that most of the clinical studies are not being shared with the public, practitioners and academia.

Over the past few years, billions of dollars' worth of tamiflu has been purchased by governments to be stockpiled in the case of a flu epidemic. This has all become subject to what is known as open data campaigns, where full transparency is being requested on the results of the clinical studies to assess efficacy and safety. The goal is to achieve appropriate and necessary independent scrutiny of data from clinical trials.

Below are some examples of agencies recommending Tamiflu without full data being researched and vetted due to the fact that the majority of the drug makers (Roche) Phase III treatment trials remain unpublished over a decade after completion.

- The World Health Organization (WHO) recommends Tamiflu, but has not vetted the Tamiflu data.

- The European Medicines Agency (EMA) approved Tamiflu, but did not review the full Tamiflu dataset.

- CDC and ECDC encourage the use and stockpiling of Tamiflu, but did not vet the Tamiflu data.

In addition to the questions raised in the reasons for stockpiling Tamiflu even when complete data is absent, leaving many to wonder the financial interests involved, Tamiflu is not side-effect free.

The most common side-effects listed on the Tamiflu packaging are nausea, vomiting and stomachache, although Roche revised the Tamiflu patient information warning that it can cause hallucinations, delirium or abnormal behavior, which sometimes 'results in fatal outcomes'.

Back in 2008, the FDA started reviewing reports of abnormal behavior and disturbing brain effects in more than 1,800 children who had taken Tamiflu. The symptoms included convulsions, delirium and delusions. In Japan, five deaths were reported in children under 16 as a result of such neurological or psychiatric problems. Seven adult deaths have also been attributed to Tamiflu, due to its neuropsychiatric effect. According to a 2009 study, more than half of children taking Tamiflu experience side effects such as nausea and nightmares.

As you can see, for a drug that is recommended and prescribed so easily, and even stockpiled to be handed out in the masses, one has to ask, why is the drug company who makes it not releasing the bulk of the research studies? And yes, the drug can come with some major side-effects, especially in light of the fact that there are other options in treating and preventing the flu.

Pharmaceutical Cartel Bribing Doctors

This has proven to be a huge problem from paying physicians as pitchmen to offering lavish gifts and trips to influence prescriber's habits. In 2012, what is now the largest criminal fraud settlement ever to come out of the pharmaceutical industry, GlaxoSmithKline (GSK) pleaded guilty and agreed to pay $1 billion in criminal fines and $2 billion in civil fines following a nine-year federal investigation into its activities- a $3 billion windfall.

When I got into pharmacy it was all about free pens and catered lunches as a motivating reason to sit down and hear a drug salesman's spiel, although as you will see, GSK up the ante big time on such 'educational influence.'

GlaxoSmithKline (GSK) was fined $3 billion after admitting bribing doctors and encouraging the prescription of unsuitable antidepressants to children. In what turned out to be a network of 49,000 doctors essentially on GSK's "payroll," it was found that the company encouraged sales reps in the United States to miss-sell three drugs to doctors while providing lavished hospitality and kickbacks on those who agreed to write extra prescriptions. Here are some of the actions that led to them getting in such hot water.

- About $600,000 a year was given to district sales representatives for entertainment, including regular golf lessons, Nascar racing days, fishing trips, and baseball and basketball tickets.

- Paxil, the anti-depressant which was only approved for adults – was promoted as suitable for children and teenagers by the company despite trials that showed it was ineffective. Children and teenagers are only treated with antidepressants in exceptional circumstances due to an increased risk of suicide, thus GSK influencing such off labeled prescribing which was even against what evidence based studies have shown was going way over the line.

- In the case of bribery, psychiatrists and their partners were flown to five-star hotels, on all-expenses-paid trips where speakers, paid up to $2,500 to attend, gave presentations on the drugs.

- GSK held eight lavish three-day events in 2000 and 2001 at hotels in Puerto Rico, Hawaii and Palm Springs, California, to promote the drug to doctors for unapproved use. Those who attended were given $750, free board and lodging and access to activities including snorkeling, golf, deep-sea fishing, rafting, glass-bottomed boat rides, hot-air balloon rides and, on one trip, a tour of the Bacardi rum distillery, all paid for by GSK.

- The popular TV and radio host, Dr. Drew, was involved with their popular anti-depressant Wellbutrin. The prosecution said the company paid $275,000 to Dr. Drew Pinsky, who hosted a popular radio show, to promote the drug on his program, in particular for unapproved uses – GSK claimed it could treat weight gain, sexual dysfunction, ADHD and bulimia.

- Sales representatives set up "Operation Hustle" to promote the drug to doctors, including trips to Jamaica, Bermuda and one talk coinciding with the annual Boston Tall Ships flotilla. Speakers were paid up to $2,500 for a one-hour presentation up to three times a day earning far more than they did working in their practices. One speaker, Dr. James Pradko, was paid nearly $1.5 million by GSK over three years to speak about the drug. He also produced a DVD funded by the company, which was claimed to be independent. It was shown more than 900 times to doctors. The hope was that doctors would be persuaded to prescribe the drug to patients over its rivals.

- Advair is GSK's block buster asthma inhaler. The company pushed the drug as the ultimate answer for tackling asthma, saying it should be the drug of choice for treating all cases. However, it had been approved only for treating severe cases, as other drugs were more suitable for mild asthma. GSK published material calling mild asthma a "myth" in an attempt to boost sales, according to the prosecution.

And just so you know this is not an isolated issue amongst GSK, this is a wide spread problems which continues today.

The folks over at propublica.org have put together an addition to their website, Dollars for Docs, http://projects.propublica.org/docdollars/ which identifies the enormity of the problem. ProPublica's Dollars for Docs database includes more than $2 billion in payments from 15 drug-makers basically enlisting doctors as a sales force, for promotional speaking, research, consulting, travel, meals and related expenses from 2009 to 2012. Payouts to hundreds of thousands physicians are now included.

Here are some other examples of drug company indiscretions which made headlines over the last few years:

- In 2012, Pfizer agreed to pay $60 million to settle allegations without admitting wrongdoing that it had long maintained a system of bribing doctors in eight countries to prescribe its drugs.

- In April 2011, Johnson & Johnson took responsibility for the bribing charges it self-reported in 2007 that its employees in Greece, Poland and Romania violated the law by bribing doctors to induce them to buy and use the company's drugs and devices.

- According to a lawsuit against pharmaceutical giant Bristol-Myers Squibb Co., doctors classified as "high prescribers" received trips to basketball camps, free concert tickets, autographed basketball merchandise, liquor, golf outings, and other rewards. Court documents show that as early as 1999, Bristol-Myers has been providing training literature for their drug reps advocating the use of incentives to prompt more prescriptions from doctors.

- TAP Pharmaceutical Products, had been charged with giving doctors ski trips to Aspen, Colorado and golf outings to Scottsdale, Arizona and Santa Barbara, California. Money that was disguised as "educational grants" was money that was actually used to pay bar tabs at cocktail parties for doctors.

False and Manipulated Studies

One of the biggest challenges and examples of deceit and lack of responsibility on the case of medical providers is in the area of evidence based medicine, essentially having a published study to back up a claim, whether it's a drug, nutritional supplement, or medical device.

Laughingly it seems a lot of practitioners feel that if it's in a study, then it must be true, although as you will soon see, this could be a gross misinterpretation of facts.

In 2009, it was shown that ghostwriters paid by a pharmaceutical company played a major role in producing 26 scientific papers backing the use of hormone replacement therapy in women, suggesting that the level of hidden industry influence on medical literature is broader than previously known.

I want to make clear, this is not to put down hormone replacement therapy, in fact, this was related to the drug company Wyeth and their blockbuster drug Premarin and Prempro, which are actually estrogen replacement from pregnant horses as well as progestin, not bio-identical progesterone.

The articles, published in medical journals between 1998 and 2005, emphasized the benefits and de-emphasized the risks of taking hormones to protect against maladies like aging skin, heart disease and dementia. That supposed medical consensus benefited Wyeth, the pharmaceutical company that paid a medical communications firm to draft the papers, as sales of its hormone drugs, called Premarin and Prempro, soared to nearly $2 billion in 2001.

Keep in mind, part of these articles deemphasized the risks, and in 2002 the Women's Health Initiative Study, a huge federal study, was halted using these medications after it was discovered that menopausal women who took certain hormones had an increased risk of invasive breast cancer, heart disease and stroke.

Remember the GSK charges mentioned above? You might find it interesting to know that fraudulent study writing was involved as well as the examples below point-out:

- GSK also paid for articles on its drugs to appear in medical journals and "independent" doctors were hired by the company to promote the treatments, according to court documents.

- GSK also published an article in a medical journal that miss-stated the Paxil's safety for children, despite the journal asking several times to change the wording. Copies of the misleading article were given to sales representatives to pass on to doctors in the hope that it would secure more business.

- Despite knowing that three trials had failed to prove its effectiveness on children, Glaxo published a report entitled "Positioning Paxil in the adolescent depression market – getting a head start."

- A study of 25 people using Wellbutrin for eight weeks was pushed by a public relations firm hired by GSK, generating headlines including "Bigger than Viagra? It sounds too good to be true: a drug to help you stop smoking, stay happy and lose weight" and "Now That is a Wonder Drug."

- When a GSK-funded doctor refused to remove safety concerns about the drug from an article he was writing, GSK removed his funding.

As you can see this prescription based medical system has not been designed to be an even playing field for those seeking the truth as well as any potential benefits and safety concerns they might have with prescription medications. Although I am encouraged to see that it seems a veil has been lifted and many of these issues are coming to the forefront with greater transparency.

Now let's take a look at how in fact there is a growing consciousness and drive towards integrative and holistic care, even from the Pharma side of things. It might only be monetarily driven, it might only be a continued form of crony capitalism and not conscious capitalism, although this is why we can make our own decisions on who to support.

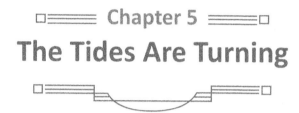

Chapter 5

The Tides Are Turning

People are looking for alternative and complementary solutions, while many others are completely opting out of this relatively young, but archaic system of western medicine. People now realize that the western form of health care does not offer unlimited health; it is not about adding life to years and years to life. This system is about keeping you just alive (or sick) enough to soak your funds and sell you more drugs.

We have a lot of things working against our health: toxins from the environment, increasing stress, declining economies, and the medical system itself. Understand though, this is all surmountable for a lifetime of vibrant health.

Following, I will address what I see as a symptomatic assessment, the main classes of drugs and disease states treated from the pharmacy counter, the divers of sick care and how they are stealing our nation's health, bankrupting the participant's at an unsustainable rate- and what you can do not to become one of the statistics mentioned earlier in the book.

The tides are now turning, we are seeing a growing amount of people opting out of the failed experiment, taking health into their own hands and becoming their own best advocate for health. They are doing their own research, they are asking more questions, and they are seeking the best practitioners and relying on them as advisors, while still realizing the ultimate responsibility lies in their own hands.

This is a patient driven movement, and it is not a fad. Integrative care is fast becoming main-stream medicine with patients asking for more solutions, and practitioners seeking opportunities to expand their practices. In 2012 alone we have seen Proctor and Gamble purchase New Chapter Vitamins, GSK announce they are creating a Traditional Chinese Medicine facility, and Nestlé Health Science and the pharmaceutical and healthcare group Chi-Med, agree to form a 50/50 joint venture to be named Nutrition Science Partners Limited (NSP). Additionally, institutes of higher education have thrown their hat into the ring with the University of South Florida offering their masters in metabolic medicine in conjunction with the Fellowship for Anti-aging and Regenerative Medicine.

This is where this book is going to take you, and even a few steps further. I find myself sharing this information every day with my clients, and often I get a look of disbelief upon the realization that their health has been the target by the pharmaceutical industry. It's called disease care; where people are kept just sick enough to be treated though a merry-go-round of drugs and tests, while never really addressing the true issues at hand.

If someone was to ask me, what are the most important things which I need to know to live a vibrant and healthy life…this is what I would tell them. And interestingly enough, if someone was then to ask me, what are the biggest untruths and lies of our medical system- they would be the same.

Part II:

HIDDEN TRUTHS AND SIMPLE STEPS TOWARDS HEALTH

"Once you make a decision, the universe conspires to make it happen"

- Ralph Waldo Emerson

What I would like to do now is to identify some of the major challenges to people's health, and how the conventional model is not necessarily healing people, but instead has them essentially tread water and in many ways slowly regress or even die way too soon. These are based on some of the most common prescriptions, as well as common disease states and symptoms which people complain of.

It is important to understand that much of this is a gradual conditioning process to the point where I see people who have forgotten what it feels like to feel great. And as people are realizing this, the exciting thing is that they are looking for options, alternatives and solutions, so this is what I will share with you as well.

I want you to look at health in a holistic manner, not as isolated systems, but how everything works together and can affect other systems. Health is multi-dimensional, a summation of mind, body, emotions and spirit, so in this section we will address the major issues, in a holistic manner. In the following sections we will talk about how to wrap it all together to attain abundant, vibrant health, as well as to provide some of my favorite resources to healing.

I will now be highlighting the most impactful areas where I believe people's health is being failed. In each section I will share with you the conventional modes of treatment, and then the alternative or complementary options.

You will see that in many of the alternative and complementary options I speak about nutritional supplements. Where I am a big supporter of quality nutritional supplements and take many supplements on a daily basis myself, my ultimate goal is not for people to be popping pills all day long. There is still a deeper level of health which we can attain and this falls within the mind-body, stress relieving techniques, and eating whole, real foods.

Everyone is individual and unique in regards to their needs. Someone who lives a relatively stress free life, eats whole organic foods and spends time supporting the mind-body, does not fall into fear and worry, exercises or 'moves' in an enjoyable fun way every day, has rewarding relationships and finds outlets for their creativity can probably get by with little to no additional supplements at all.

For someone who is knee deep in the culture of stress, does not eat the best diet, is working a job which does not support professional or personal values, might not get adequate sleep every night, and does not have the opportunity or ability to eat all organic, all the time, well, than nutritional supplementation might be needed.

I personally would rather see someone using natural medicines opposed to chemical and synthetic for many of the reasons I have already spoken about. What I encourage everyone to do is to dig deeper, get into the root of your health, understand the benefits of separating from your ego, recognize the power of the mind-body, and realize that your outer being and outer health is merely a mirror to your inner health.

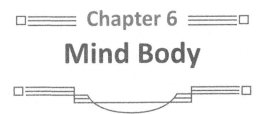

Chapter 6

Mind Body

There exists a place in every person, a place that is free from disease, never feels pain, and is ageless and never dies- when we journey to this place, limitation's we commonly accept simply cease to exist- they're not even a possibility -this is the place called perfect health. Stepping into this realm, no matter how brief these visits may be, can bring profound transformation and healing, in this state of true mind body spirit connects and all previous assumptions about ordinary existence disappear and we experience a higher truly ideal reality

- Deepak Chopra

As a pharmacist, you might find it odd on how much credit I give the mind-body, although I believe it is the one major factor for all areas of our existence, which we must give regular attention to. I am about to show you what the mind body really means; how it can lead to illness, and how you can use it to support your health. I will be transitioning from how mind body medicine has been categorically excluded from conventional medicine, share with you some examples, give you some hard science and then transition into the metaphysical.

When we think of our health, we often just look at our physical bodies. I would like you to look at your body as a vessel which you use to experience life, to influence others, impact the world around you, and to attain the best life that you can for you and your loved ones. As you will see, this physical representation, our vehicle to get through life is driven by something deeper, and this is the connection of the mind, body and spirit. Even where someone might have great limitations in their physical body or the material world, the immutable truth is that everyone is an unlimited spiritual being, and it is the connection of the mind body that allows people to change their particular condition or experience one of few limitations.

We live in a universe made up of energy and surrounded by energy. Because we all share in the universal energy that unifies us, no compartment of life is shut off from another. The smallest parts of life and matter reflect properties of the universe as a whole. Physicist David Bohm called this the holographic universe: *every aspect of our lives has a reflection in every other aspect.* This means how you do health is how you do life. Our relationship with health is a metaphor for our relationship with all forms of energy: money, time, enjoyment, creativity, relationships- everything.

Let's suppose our health, and for that matter, our reality, is divided into two parts. One aspect is the physical reality. This is the physical representation of your health; how you look, how you feel, your lab tests, your weight, and diseases or physical symptoms you might acquire. In this realm, energy is coalesced into objects that have form, density, and size. These are the tangibles, anything you can see, taste, feel, or smell.

The physical is based on impermanence; things grow, die, change form and shape, and are replaced. Your physical body is a perfect example, from cradle to grave, birth, growth, changes in age and ultimately death. To move or change objects in this domain you have to focus energy on them. For instance, if you want to build muscle the most benefit will come from physically adding stress to your muscles to make them stronger and force them to grow. (You will learn later that 'just thinking about it' does have a particular application though in activating the same areas of the brain as physical application does.)

Then there is the metaphysical reality. In this realm, energy has not been solidified into form. It is free flowing and unbounded. Whatever exists here is intangible and cannot be measured by the usual physical means. Elements in the metaphysical reality are immune to the law of impermanence. As we experience this realm consciously and unconsciously, through our imagination, visions, emotions and intentions, we realize this is where the seeds of our health, happiness, wealth, and relationships are created.

We interact with this plane all the time, knowingly and unknowingly. Health comes as the result of the combined contribution of what has begun and nurtured in the metaphysical realm and then brought to life and grown in the physical domain.

Psychosomatic Medicine

Have you ever heard a doctor or someone say "it's all in your head"? Well, an illness might be, it might be in your head, your emotions, or embedded deep into your beliefs, but this does not mean it is not a real physical problem- nor does it mean that you have a psychological disorder either. On the contrary, it is a very real thing, and thoughts and emotions can influence the development of an illness, so let's take a look at the history of psychosomatic (aka mind body) medicine in our society. Incidentally, I will be using the terms psychosomatic and mind body interchangeably.

Psychosomatic medicine specifically refers to physical disorders of the mind body, disorders that may appear to be purely physical, but which have their origin in unconscious emotions, a very different and extremely important medical matter.

This, like other areas of our health and the health care system, has been systematically hijacked over the years. The DSM (Diagnostic and Statistical Manual of Mental Disorders) is basically the "psychiatry bible" and scripts "standard of care" while at the same time deciding what is reimbursable (or labeled as a disease) by insurance. The board of the American Psychiatric Association makes changes and approvals to the DSM and in what has probably been one of the biggest actions to castrate the recognition of mind-body medicine has been the removal of the term psychosomatic from recent editions of the DSM. As Dr. John Sarno, M.D. puts it in his book *The Divided Mind*, *"One might as well eliminate the word infection from medical dictionaries."*

I personally came upon the power of mind body medicine in my own professional career and personal life which shows a great significance to the power of conditioning. I grew up in a family of "bad backs". My back used to "go out" on me. It would stiffen up at the result of me doing something so simple, such as picking up a sock.

This would come and go for years until it became a hardened identity within me (which I like to call the identity of illness). After going to a chiropractor, X-rays shown that I had "degenerative disc disease." I rehabbed, I stretched, I weight trained. This went on for years and finally I found my way to an orthopedic surgeon. This trip to the surgeon gave me what I was looking to hear for a long time, the recommendation of back surgery. Sounds crazy right? One might think that my relief to hear the recommendation of surgery was based on the hope that my back pain would finally be eradicated, although I believe it was a deeper trip down the rabbit hole of my identity to the illness in some unconscious twisted way; it was further helping me identify with who I thought I was.

Surgery was a "success" and after about a month I was cleared to resume life (admittedly by my physician, earlier than usual). Living in a ski town as we were at the time, resuming life often means getting back on to your snowboard or ski's, and this was the case for me.

(Incidentally, my back surgeon, became quite well-known for a life-experience of dying, coming back to life, and being touched by God, and now in addition to her practice, continues to spread her story and message in helping others. I encourage you to read her book, *To Heaven and Back, as* this will provide further impact on the power of our spiritual / non-physical realm.*)*

When the ski season came to an end, Amy and I then took a spring vacation to Costa Rica, traveling throughout the country, experiencing their roads around pot holes, cramped airplane rides, surfing, and trekking; all this and not a twinge of pain. Then, vacation ended, and it was back at work. I had resistance about going back into the pharmacy that I had left run on auto pilot for two weeks. I walked into the pharmacy, caught up on what I had missed, and Wham! - Muscle spasm and sciatica down my legs; it literally took my breath away. What the heck! I thought, they cut the protruding discs out, this shouldn't be happening.

Do you see what happened? I was so ingrained to the belief and identity of having a bad back that surgery did not alleviate the issue. It initially allowed it to lay dormant. Then a measure of stress via mental and emotional aspects eventually presented itself, it triggered the cascade of events which brought me back to ground zero. Regardless of the surgery, regardless of the stretching and strengthening, a conditioned belief combined with the control issues that represented via the lower back, and I was blind-sided before I knew what had hit me.

After coming to this realization, my life is no longer limited by issues of back pain; I never alter my activities due to it. If in fact, if my back or neck stiffens up, I realize that it most likely is a combination of a mind and body element. John Sarno calls this TMS (tension myositis syndrome), which in basic terms is a build-up of tension and emotions in a physical form. I personally feel that this plays a very big role in the majority of chronic pain cases on one level or another, and looking at in a more holistic approach can help make a positive impact.

What I do is immediately go into some EFT (Emotional Freedom Technique), aka "tapping" which you will learn about in section III, and maybe a visit to the chiropractor, and by the next day I am all better.

Science- Not Unicorns and Rainbows

I know what some of you might be thinking- *"this whole mind body thing sounds great, but is it real?"*, or *"this is not based on science, prove it!"* or how about, *"this kind of thinking is dangerous, filling people's head with false hope."*

And in the conventional medical role, the FDA would have a field day with some of this stuff, but what I would like you to do is approach it with an open mind, maybe suspend any disbelief one might have, do not stop any program your doctor has you on, and enjoy the read.

The fact is, it is very real, and sometimes one must suspend their disbelief to let go and get past false programming and conditioning that they have held onto so strongly for so long. Shortly we will get into the control that the ego mind has over us, but first, let's look at some science.

The view of traditional health and cell biology is that physical molecules control biology and that genetics control our behavior and health- basically our genetics control our life and we have no say in the matter. This is false and it has been proven to be false by the work of Dr. Bruce Lipton PHD, author of *The Biology of Belief*, where his work shows that genes and DNA do not control our biology; instead that DNA is controlled by signals from outside the cell, including the energetic messages emanating from our positive and negative thoughts, and that it is the quality of energy itself that controls bodily function and health.

Dr. Lipton has been a pioneer in applying the principles of quantum physics to the field of cellular biology and his work focuses on the mechanisms through which genes can be turned on and off by environmental signals and energy in the form of thoughts, feelings, and emotions which than affect our biology and outwardly our physical health.

In his groundbreaking work, Dr. Lipton shows that human beings can control gene activity and even rewrite their genes by focusing on their thoughts and beliefs. Change the thought environment in which cells are submerged in, the cells will change and so will our behavior; thus our bodies can be changed as a result of us retraining our thinking. Dr. Lipton also shows how even our most firmly held beliefs can be changed, which means that we have the power to reshape our lives. We now know the brain is what controls our chemistry and our minds control our brain, and adopting new beliefs is not only spiritually and emotionally comforting, but vitally important to our physical health.

Facts reveal for example, that genes do not control cancer or heart disease. Cells, it turns out, are intelligent. They read our environmental and mental and emotional stimuli and adjust their behavior. They translate information into a biochemical 'awareness' that regulates their activity. They eat, excrete and communicate intelligently to exchange information. They are controlled by signals coming from our own thinking and emotions, from the food we ingest, toxins in our environment, and the exercise which we do and don't do. Experiments conducted by Dr. Lipton reveal that the outer layer of a cell is the organic equivalent of a computer chip, and the cell's equivalent of a brain. So in fact, it is the influence that is placed upon the membrane of the cells which influence how the cells act, how healthy they live and how healthy they die.

Let me give you another example in the field of nutria-genomics, which is essentially the influence of ones genes by dietary supplements and foods. Polyphenols are the active constituents of green tea, pine bark, grape seed, pomegranate, turmeric, and berries such as raspberries and blueberries. Polyphenols are often noted and cited for their antioxidant activity, although research is showing how these compounds orchestrate healthy cellular communication and gene expression to support nearly every aspect of health- they can turn on the good genes and turn off the bad.

So as you can see, it's more than mind over matter, or coincidence or luck. The most advanced foremost research stands behind the theory that our environment, our thoughts and beliefs do in fact have the ability to influence our state of health, good or bad. And I am not saying that if you change your thinking and environment than your health will change immediately and miraculously. This is a process and health is a commitment.

The Self Image- Your Secret Weapon To Health

"Nothing splendid has ever been achieved except by those who dared believe that something inside them was superior to circumstance." - Bruce Barton

Back in the 1960's, Dr. Maxwell Maltz began to write about self-image in his ground breaking book, *Psycho-Cybernetics*, which has become the basis to the self-help movement of the past fifty years.

By understanding your self-image and by learning to modify it and manage it to suit your purposes, you gain empowerment over your situation, including your health. Each and every one of us has a mental picture of ourselves, who we believe we are. For some this is an active or even proactive conscious recognition, for others it might be purely under the influence of the subconscious.

Our self-image has been sculpted around our thoughts and beliefs about ourselves, past experiences, what we have told ourselves, what society and others have told us, our successes and our failures. In short, you will "act like" and enjoy the limitless or limited aspects of health and life of the sort of person you conceive yourself to be.

Dr. Maxwell Maltz writes in his book, Psycho-Cybernetics:

"When we experience expansive emotions of happiness, self-confidence, and success, we enjoy more life. And to the degree that we inhibit our abilities, frustrate our God-given talents, and allow ourselves to suffer anxiety, fear, self-condemnation and self-hate, we literally choke off the life force available to us and turn our back on the gift that our Creator has made. To the degree that we deny the gift of life, we embrace death."

It's the same with health, when we allow a false sense of self to exist, when we succumb to the thoughts and emotions of anxiety, fear, and limiting beliefs, we deny ourselves the gift of health, and embrace disease.

Ego Driven Medicine

*"The Death of The Ego Will Be The Beginning
of Your Real Life"* - Unknown

Imagine a world where all children had high self-esteem and adults were not victims of their ego.

A poor self-image is a critical reason why people do not obtain the health, wealth, and happiness that they are searching for, and often fall victim to their egos. A healthy self-image is the anecdote to an uncontrolled ego. This in fact is where the line exists between confidence (a positive result of healthy self-esteem) and ego.

The ego hijacks your self-image. The ego blurs ones interpretation of a given situation versus the facts. The ego separates one from self. A common habit of many with a low self-image or where ego is in charge is to interpret the words and deeds of others as though they were intended as a personal assault when in fact this is often not the case. The same goes for the words one says about themselves, the negative self-talk that actually comes from their ego and not from the truth. Most issues of low self-image are projected by your ego, and then take residence within your thoughts and emotions.

Only you can build up your self-image, and only your ego can tear it down. The ego wants you to see your body, your health, your being, as separate, disconnected from self. The uncontrolled ego is responsible for more challenges to one's mind and body from practicing self-pity, blaming, negative self-talk, acting out of fear and grasping the identity of illness, to not being able to let go of certain issues thus moving forward, to self-sabotaging oneself on a path to wellness.

When the ego is in control, we in some way choose some sort of insane belief about ourselves, our body, our health, and therefore the ego uses our body and health for the its own benefit. When you perceive your body negatively (physically ill, addicted, overweight, not good enough, etc.) you've chose to take your ego's perception out on your body, thereby strengthening the ego.

It's likely that at some point in time you have been caught up in the ego's projection of your health which is often rooted out a negative thought, emotion or judgment. Without understanding the root cause of this issue, you felt like a victim, powerless to change or take control of the situation. You might be there right now, maybe you know of a friend or a loved one going through such as situation.

When medicine experienced the shift from purpose driven healing to ego driven bottom lines, the ego became the biggest roadblock to people's wellbeing. As the saying goes "as above, so below" this has become a virus within the conventional western style of medicine, trickling down to the law makers, insurers, practitioner's and patients. When there is a system created out of an ego driven energy, optimal healing will not occur.

Let's take a look at some examples where the ego might take control through your thoughts, emotions and actions leading to disempowerment of your health.

1) You blame others for your state of health.

2) You associate yourself with your disease or diagnosis, falling into the identity of illness.

3) You have a hard time of letting go of issues in your life, perceptions where you feel you have been harmed and keep recycling these issues into your life.

4) You feel afraid to question or ask for an alternative to what your doctor orders.

5) You compare your health or your body to others.

6) You get offended at someone's actions or words intended as support, but you perceive it as an attack in regards to your health or the health of a loved one.

7) You react out of fear about a lab test that "tags" you with a disease, which is merely an imbalance represented by symptoms which can be brought into balance.

8) You judge others by projecting your views of health on others.

9) You catch yourself emotionally binge eating, irrationally starving yourself or falling victim to some sort of negative food behavior.

10)　You use your body to reinforce external qualities about yourself such as flaunting your body to feel good about yourself, using your looks to gets something or gain an advantage, or even to receive positive reinforcement from other people.

11)　You regularly swim in the sea of self-pity which keeps you stuck in your perceived condition without working your way out.

And I understand, at times it's difficult not to fall victim to the egos projections, although as you can see there are numerous ways the ego can get between the true you and true health.

ENERGY

"Everything is energy and that's all there is to it. Match the frequency of the reality you want, and you cannot help but get that reality. It can be no other way, this is not philosophy; this is physics."

-Albert Einstein

As one of the greatest minds of our time points out, everything is energy and you can change your reality…it's science, this is not philosophy, and I believe it to be the same about one's health. So let's get into what I believe is one of the most powerful tools for your health, well, your entire existence, and how it is so underutilized in conventional medicine.

As we now move into the finer points of the mind body continuum, I would like you to look at your body as vibrational. Right now are you vibrating high or vibrating low? Can you think back to a time when you were operating on a lower vibrational frequency? Or when an event seemed to knock you down? Maybe it was hearing that a loved one was not coming to visit for the holidays, or maybe you did not qualify for a mortgage, or get into the college you wanted.

Now do the opposite. Think about a time when you were vibrating at a higher frequency, something many would call being in "state" or "the zone." Everything flows perfectly, you feel great, and nothing can knock you down. This could have been your wedding day or feeling great on a particular vacation exploring new areas you have never seen, or maybe it was getting an A+ on a particular project or receiving a raise. Maybe there was a time when an incident shifted you from a lower vibrating frequency to a higher one? Receiving an unexpected check in the mail, maybe a letter from an old friend you were not expecting for whom you have not heard from in a while.

This is a big part of how we grow, how we fall ill, and how we heal. It's all about energy. In asking ourselves, what creates one's health, we should instead ask, what creates anything? And the answer is- energy.

Energy is everywhere, there is energy in everything. Thoughts are energy, beliefs are energy, emotions are energy, our actions are energy, and remember as Dr. Bruce Lipton has discovered, it's the quality of energy that matters.

Energy, Matter, and Your Health

This all stems from science described in Einstein's Theory of Relativity. In the general definition of relativity, Einstein shows that matter and energy actually mold the shape of space and the flow of time.

The Law of Thermodynamics states; "energy can neither be created nor destroyed, it can only be changed from one form to another", and one of those forms is matter. Matter is created from energy all the time (growth) and transformed (change back into energy) through decomposition, and then molded into shape again.

Everything in this physical existence has been created from energy, often in the source of an originating thought. Thoughts create things (things are accumulation of matter), and this includes you and your health. If your health is comprised of energy; the energy of belief, thought, emotion, and action, then you have the ability to transform your state of health.

Universal energy is creative, universal energy is based on transformation. The universe is constantly creating and transforming old to new, that is what it does. The universe has abundance of energy to allow you to transform exactly what you would like in life and this holds true to your health. The universe does not know lack. Thus a lack of good health is actually the same energy transformed to abundance of ill health, or disease- the quality of the energy changes. Lack is only a perception, a perception which is further backed and influenced by thoughts, beliefs and emotions.

When I say "The Universe" it can mean many things; Holy Spirit, source, God, whatever you wish, but the thing to realize is that we are all connected to it and we are mirrors of it. As the saying goes, *as above, so below,* we are creative and transforming beings ourselves, although it is up to us to decide which direction we want our creative and transforming energies to flow.

Now let's look at this from a metaphysical point of view. Marianne Williamson, best-selling author and teacher of *A Course in Miracles* has said:

> *"Every thought is a cause that produces an effect. According to A Course in Miracles, every thought we think creates form on some level. If your mind is in a loving place-if thoughts are a high, divine vibration- your experience will reflect that. If your mind is in a fearful place-if your thoughts are of a lower, dense vibration-your experience will reflect that. The way to change the nature of your experience is to change the nature of your thoughts."*

Sounds a lot like Dr. Bruce Lipton's work, doesn't it? -Metaphysics meets science.

If this is true, which I believe it is, then the problem is things such as fear, worry, and dense, negative thoughts can lead to physical issues of disease. Any disease has a manifestation in the mind-body, which is further influenced by a disempowered model of health.

Often what is needed is a shift in perception and attention to influence and manifest the energy and health that you wish. A Course in Miracles identifies a miracle as just that, a shift in perception. A shift in perception from fear to love- whatever ones perception will then have influence on ones thoughts, beliefs, and ultimately actions, thus addressing health in the physical.

Life Force-Qi

"We are not human beings having a spiritual experience; we are spiritual beings having a human experience."

— Pierre Teilhard de Chardin

…Yet our western system of medicine focuses our life and our health only on the physical.

In traditional Chinese culture, qì (also chi or ch'i) is an active principle forming part of any living thing; qi is the flow of energy, otherwise referred to as life-force. Where qi is the central underlying principle in Traditional Chinese Medicine, concepts similar to qi can be found in many cultures, for example, Prana in Vedic philosophy, Mana in Hawaiian culture, Lüng in Tibetan Buddhism, and Vital energy in Western philosophy.

Qi plays a very big role in many traditional healing systems across the globe with the belief that disease results at the stagnation, or blocking of qi. This flow of life force energy is the basis to modalities of medicine such as acupuncture, acupressure and Qigong, the practice of working with life energy via moving meditation of aligning breath, movement, and awareness for exercise, and healing.

When one begins to focus on not just the quality of their energy, but the flow of their energy, recognizing an ancient spiritual practice applied to modern day living, miraculous results in regards to one's health can result. We will get into more of this in the resource section when we speak about qigong, although benefits include; enhanced creativity, immune system support, pain management, vitality, increased energy, reduced stress and more.

Attraction and Expansion

"Worry is prayer for chaos." - Unknown

You know the saying, "be careful what you wish for?" Consider a 'wish' in this case to be those unguarded thoughts in the forms of worry and fear that can fly around in one's head. Basically what we are saying is that what you focus your attention on, while adding corresponding and congruent emotions, you can attract and it will expand in your life- good and bad.

For me this was the conditioning of seeing everyone in my family having bad backs. I saw it so often, heard words spoken and experienced situations around being victims to back pain that it became my reality. I have seen this in numerous clients.

One example was a female in her 30-'s who opted for a voluntary double mastectomy when she was diagnosed with breast cancer. As she told her story, she said, "After seeing my aunt go through breast cancer, I always said, if I get breast cancer, I will choose to have a mastectomy." Not to be void of empathy, although my thought was, "You got what you feared and put your attention towards." The ordeal of seeing a loved one go through illness is challenging enough when your main intention is for their best interest.

It is important to understand that our genetics and experiences are not a life sentence, they do not write our story, and as Dr. Lipton has pointed out, our genes can be turned on and off by environmental signals-including thoughts, feelings and emotions from outside the cell.

So let's now get into how we can influence what we want for ourselves through the law of attraction and the law of expansion.

These laws state that whatever you choose to focus your attention upon will expand and you will attract it. The laws of attraction and expansion are what direct the energy that molds our lives. Now, I am not saying all you have to do is focus on something and it will appear. What I am reminding you that this is physics as Einstein states in his quote:

"Everything is energy and that's all there is to it. Match the frequency of the reality you want, and you cannot help but get that reality. It can be no other way, this is not philosophy; this is physics."

When ones thoughts and emotions are congruent with the laws of attraction and expansion, this is what it takes for the frequency match he was speaking about.

Our current health care system, for the most part, chooses to focus on issues of lack, fear, and illness. Think about medications, they are "anti" everything; antibiotics, anti-inflammatories, antihistamines, etc. So what do we get a nation full of? You guessed it, lack of abundant health, fear of ill health, flat out anti-health and materialization and expansion of illness. Can you imagine where we would be if we were taught to focus on health fortifying issues and solutions that worked with and not against our bodies?

Your state of health today is the direct result of where you have focused your energy and attention in the past. Your future state of health will be determined by where you focus your attention and energy now. If you desire abundant health in your future, you should focus on abundant aspects of your health today.

So, whether it is the thoughts that you think, the words that you speak, or the actions that you take, I ask you to start focusing on what you want to manifest within your health. I am not claiming that any of this is a formula for spontaneous healing, although I do believe in the body's inherent ability to heal when everything can fall into place.

Physical Energy Matching

We know that our minds can change our bodies and our behavior, although can our bodies change our minds? Science has shown that it is possible; let me share with you a few examples.

Try modeling. Begin to model parts of your life, no matter how minute, directed towards exactly what you want. Modeling is another form of energy matching (remember Einstein's quote). Modeling has been taught through the system of high performance, Neurolinguistic Programming (NLP), and proven successful time and time again.

What you do is you envision the perfect you, or even someone who you admire with particular values. Visualize what you would look like, how you would feel, what thoughts would you think, what level of energy would you have, what would you be doing? What values and beliefs would you have, what would people say about you, how would you envision yourself walking down the street?

Or, maybe you have a hero or someone you admire for a particular reason. In this case you can take on their characteristics, work ethic, even hobbies. You see this all the time with successful athletes when they say who they once looked up to, and often they "magically" acquire the same physical talents and attributes. You can take a number of people you admire, maybe the athletic prowess of one, the shrewd business sense of someone else, and the compassion of another. It's all about the values you want to see outwardly present themselves in you.

Here's the kicker, you want to be consistent with this, because when it comes down to it, an unhealthy self-image can play sabotage if left unattended. There is something known as the snap-back affect. If deep down your self-image is not an energy match, if you do not believe you are a match for this energy transplant, like a rubber form, you will inevitably snap-back to what you believe yourself to be.

Fortunately through the science of power dynamics and Power Posing, we know that you can "fake it until you become it" in just a few minutes each day. I will be delving more into power posing and this science in section three, although the research that Amy J.C. Cuddy, a social psychologist and professor at Harvard Business School, and colleagues have done shows that by tiny tweaks in your physical posture your body can change your mind in powerful ways.

What makes this science ever so more compelling is that Amy has proven this in her own life, against the beliefs of the conventional medical profession that the physical actions you take can in fact influence and change your mind, beliefs and outcomes. A highly intelligent undergrad, Amy was in a car accident which left her with a brain trauma, she lost significant I.Q. points where her physicians suggested that she probably was not going to finish college. Amy decided the doctors were wrong and decided she did not have to accept things as they appeared to be, and her continual accomplishments in academia and life have proven her choice correct.

Power posing gives us another amazing tool for simple shifts in perception and action, to lead to the major changes in health and life that we wish.

Science has proven that when you are happy you smile, although if you are forced to smile by putting a pencil between your teeth, you also become happy even if you were not happy to begin with. Taking this bit of information and after studying the traits of high performance individuals, Amy set off to see if you can actually change your physical position to one of power, to feel more powerful.

Through her research Amy realized that high powered producers, executives, leaders, even primates and animals, were more assertive, confident, and optimistic, they think more abstractly and take more risks. These same traits also coalesce with hormones in our body. Our hormones are chemical messengers, hormones affect how we act and react, and the best leaders have higher testosterone and lower cortisol- this is across the evolutionary spectrum, from primates to people. By partaking in high power poses for just 2 minutes, someone can raise their testosterone 20%, decrease their cortisol 25%, and by partaking in low power poses, someone will decrease their testosterone by 10% and raise their cortisol by 15%. When we get to the chapter on hormones, you will understand this impact, and we will be speaking more on the science of power posing in section three.

MANIFEST YOUR HEALTH

Alright, so now let's look at how your state of health plays out like a recipe. We just talked about the ingredients; energy, quality of energy and vibration of thoughts, influences of both attraction and expansion. Now let's see how these ingredient's work together in what we call the formula for manifestation.

This formula basically transmutes intangible thought impulses of desire and attraction into its physical counterpart of health. This formula is scribed from your experiences and your life and is very unique to you. This formula is very simple. This formula is the culmination of your past and present conditioning, beliefs, thoughts, emotions, actions and habits.

We are creatures of habit; we learn by example and are influenced heavily by our environment and relationships. The influences that we have experienced and endured, especially at a young age, provide the fodder for our belief patterns.

Through the power of autosuggestion and conditioning these experiences program certain beliefs into our subconscious. These programmed beliefs will then produce our thoughts upon what we believe and perceive to be right or wrong, what is good or bad, what is important and not so important.

This culmination of thoughts will lead to a corresponding culmination of emotions. Fear based thoughts lead to fear based emotions, empowering thoughts lead to empowering emotions, see how it works? Emotions are catalysts. They are the primary power to transmute the non-physical to the physical. They are the engine that converts "nothing" into something. They are the fuel for the fire.

The emotions will now lead to actions because after all, emotions are energy in motion, e-motion. E-motions lead to our physical actions, which over time become habits and due to a repetitive nature will determine our exact state of health.

Very simply, here is the Equation to Manifestation of Health…

➡ Past & Present conditioning lead to Beliefs &Perceptions

➡ Beliefs & Perceptions lead to Thoughts

➡ Thoughts lead to Emotions

➡ Emotions lead to Actions and Habits

➡ Actions and Habits lead to further Experiences and Conditioning…

…Rinse and Repeat

Now let's break each of these parts of the formula down and look at them one by one.

PAST & PRESENT CONDITIONING

Have you ever realized that people often end up with characteristics of one of or both of their parents?

Whether it is a sense of humor, quirky habits, financial outcomes and even health and wellbeing, we have a tendency to model ourselves after what we have been influenced by.

Why do you think this is? Genetics? I will not deny, genetics may play a role in an individual's health, but a genetic trait generally will not present itself unless it is provided the environment to do so. Remember, Dr. Bruce Lipton discovered that environment can alter genetics. This is exactly why we should practice preventative health. So, yes, disease can run in the family, though we can either stack the cards in our favor or against ourselves.

Your current conditioning either comes from your childhood or overcoming your childhood. From childhood to the present, the conditioning and situations that you experience, conscious or unconscious, can have a tremendous outcome on your health.

Past conditioning is what molds our belief structure and plays a very strong role on how we perceive our reality to be. These are the words we have heard, sights we have seen, and situations that we have felt and experienced.

Present conditioning and experiences quickly become the past; this demonstrates the impact that the now has. What happened to you yesterday is continually shaping new belief structures of today, and for tomorrow.

What kind of conditioning are we speaking of?

First, the most important thing to keep in mind is that in any given situation we will absorb the experience both actively and passively, which means conditioning happens on both a conscious and subconscious level.

If you put a child in a disempowering environment such as abuse or poor eating habits, they will soak it up like a sponge. If you put a child in an empowering environment such as love or healthy eating habits, they will also soak it up like a sponge.

If a child grows up with no role model for exercise or even spending time outdoors, what do you think will carry over in exercise habits as they age? If a child grows up being rewarded with junk food, what type of conditioning of "good food" & "bad food" do you think they will have?

BELIEFS

> *"Beliefs have the power to create and the power to destroy. Human beings have the awesome ability to take any experience of their lives and create a meaning that disempowers them or one that can literally save their lives."*
>
> - Tony Robbins

Our beliefs are the core structures that are created by past and present conditioning. Beliefs are the foundational elements to everything; cultural dogma's, media influence, corporations, family conditioning, political systems, educational institutions, religions, everything!

Belief systems, whether conscious or unconscious, play an enormous role in the health, wealth, and happiness of an individual. The intensity of belief and desire plays a strong role in the outcome of our health. If deep down, you do not believe or desire to get healthy, chances are you will not, it's that simple.

No matter how wonderful the next drug is, or how brilliant a health care practitioner may be, nothing can stand up to the power of a belief in disease or not allowing oneself to get healthy and overcome that problem. The opposite of a miracle, these intense negative beliefs can bring such non-physical energy to the physical plane.

Something that goes hand in hand with belief is faith. The corner stone to a healthy belief system is faith. If you are looking to change your belief structure, maybe past conditioning has trained you to believe that you are not worthy or able to attain excellence in health, start with the power of faith.

You might find yourself in a situation where your beliefs are being challenged, and it is through the power of faith that will keep you on course. Faith frees your energy, thoughts, and emotions opening your mind and beliefs of new possibilities. Faith gives you confidence, keeps you from sinking into victimization, a position that attracts more victimization, and lifts you to positivity, which attracts more positive outcomes. Faith is responsible for energy shifts within you.

What faith is not is a free pass to give up your responsibility of taking right action through thoughts, emotions and actions. I have seen many a person feel their health is some sort of destiny, what will be, will be- this does not have to be the case.

Limiting Beliefs of Society

Society has instilled many limits on what is believed to be possible. We adopt these limits as fact while consciously and unconsciously allowing them to guide and mold our lives, from our wealth to our health to our happiness. We must realize that the only limits to our existence are the limits that we accept and place upon ourselves.

There are countless real-life stories of people overcoming their own personal or others belief to attain health and healing. Arthur Boorman is such an example. For 15 years doctors told him he would never walk unassisted again due to injuries to his legs and back he sustained from being a paratrooper in the Gulf War. This man was then resigned to a wheel chair or crutches to move around, and in doing so he gained a lot of weight, and exercise seemed impossible.

He began his quest, thinking yoga could help, and where most instructors turned him away, one in particular decided to help him on his path.

Fast forward 10 months, Arthur lost 140 pounds. Arthur is back to his vibrant healthy being, not only is he able to walk, but he can run, and regularly practices yoga like a master. And this was all after doctors told him he would never walk unassisted again- fortunately, he did not believe them.

Another incredible example is a man named Sean Stephenson who was born with osteogenesis imperfecta, commonly known as "brittle bone disease." During birth, most of his bones had been broken and due to his condition doctors warned his parents that he might not survive. He did survive, but spent much of his youth in pain, suffering broken bones and experienced the stunted growth and mobility limitations most people with this condition experience.

This would understandably resign most people to a life of limitations considering the physical and even emotional challenges one would face. Think about the challenges; what type of work could he get, would he be able to have a relationship, get married? The list goes on and Sean has overcome every one of them, fortunately, since Sean did not listen to the beliefs of doctors and society. Today Sean is happily married; he is a college graduate and licensed therapist, author, motivational speaker and successful business man.

One must realize the only true meaning any situation has is the meaning that one give's it. Essentially, one's reality is how he/she believes and perceives a situation to be.

There are probably countless instances in your life where "the reality of the situation was not what it was believed to be." The ingredients to the situation led to a "misunderstanding" of sorts. These instances are heavily influenced by the beliefs that the participants had coming into it.

Find your limiting beliefs, especially the ones relating to your health, conquer them and create the template for others to follow. Dare to tread where others have not treaded before. Prove yours and societies limiting beliefs wrong; create your own miracle.

THOUGHTS & THE MIND

"Be sure that what's on your mind right now is something you're willing to experience in your life"

- Cheryl Richardson

As you have learned in the Formula for Manifestation your thoughts stem from current and previous conditioning and beliefs. Everything around you has been created through a thought process, whether conscious or unconscious, good or bad. Your thoughts have a direct correlation to your health, happiness, and wellbeing. The greatest thing about your thoughts is that you can take immediate action to control them.

As the best-selling author, student and teacher of *A Course In Miracles*, Marianne Williamson states:

"From a metaphysical perspective, every experience begins with a thought and our experience changes when we change the thought. If we have a problem in any area- whether relationships, health, money, or anything else- the first place to look for solutions is in the nature of our thinking."

A lot of this can become hindered by the ego which we spoke about earlier. If left unchained, the ego mind can be your inner voice of negativity, and in a self-defeating sort of way, talk you out of your hopes, wishes, goals and desires.

Let's see how this all works with our conscious and subconscious mind. The primary job of our conscious mind is self-preservation and protection. The primary job of the sub-conscious is manifestation and projection. It's through the often ill-fated judgments of our conscious mind often ruled by ego which imprints messages on our sub-conscious mind that creates our conscious world.

Here is how it works…

With any impulse of thought which is repeatedly passed on to the subconscious mind, the greater chance that it is accepted and acted upon.

The subconscious mind proceeds to translate that impulse into its physical equivalent by the most practical route available.

Here is the take home. The subconscious mind makes no distinction between constructive and destructive thoughts. It works with the material that we are feeding it through our thought impulses. The subconscious mind will translate into reality a thought driven by fear just as readily as it will translate a thought driven by love.

The conscious mind acts on what it believes and perceives which as we have shown comes from past influences and experiences. The conscious mind can often lose control to the ego, which will send low energy, high negative thoughts such as the 5 most addictive drugs it dispenses; self-pity, blame, identity of illness, fear, and negative self-talk.

Thus, especially in a medical system which is not created through values and empowerment, one must work to imprint the higher energy, empowered thoughts on to its subconscious to attain positive health.

To change your health, you often have to make changes to all areas of your being and the ego does not like this. For the ego minds' judgments and decisions, it relies upon two primary tools, memory and emotion. Memories and emotions may surface at times that we have failed at something (ex- yo yo dieting), or repetitive influences and experiences of ill health. Our conscious mind perceives this as "remember how awful that was, why would you even want to consider going back there?" or "it didn't work then why would it work now?"

Here is a way to diffuse the energy out of ego generated thoughts. I learned this one from Gabrielle Bernstein's book, *May Cause Miracles*, and basically anytime you have a disempowering thought, or negative self-talk, say the following affirmation. In fact, write it down on a piece of paper and train yourself to read it each time you have a disempowering thought until it becomes a memorized and embedded reaction to your psyche.

"I forgive myself for having this thought- I choose love instead."

- Gabrielle Bernstein

EMOTIONS

"Take control of your consistent emotions and begin to consciously and deliberately reshape your daily experience of life"

- Tony Robbins

Thoughts which have been emotionalized immediately begin to translate themselves into their physical equivalent. Basically, emotions are what give thoughts the vitality of life. They are the fuel to convert the non-physical into the physical. Emotions are how we feel about ourselves, a certain thing, place, person or situation.

The more emotion or feeling you have towards something, the quicker and more efficiently it can be translated into this physical reality. This is such a powerful concept that it only behooves us to monitor our emotions, and immediately convert the non-empowering emotions to empowering emotions, thus empowering actions. The best way to analyze emotions is how you react or respond to a given situation.

If you allow yourself to react you are not taking full responsibility for yourself, your emotions, or your health. If you choose to respond, then you are acting out of full "respond-ability" and therefore put yourself in the best position for emotional empowerment and action.

Below are some examples of emotions that we see present themselves in many states of disease:

- Fear
- Frustration
- Guilt
- Anger
- Resentment

Do you ever think and react out of *fear*?

Do you ever think and react out of *frustration*?

Do you ever think and react out of *guilt*?

Do you ever think and react out of *anger*?

Do you ever think and react out of *resentment*?

These emotions, whether they are spoken, thought, or felt can act as poison in the body. They create a stress response that can dramatically influence the symptoms that you are currently experiencing in regards to any illness. For instance, if you have a bad back, when these negative emotions encompass you, does your condition worsen? What if you are dealing with digestive disorders such as irritable bowel syndrome or even the chronic pain experienced in fibromyalgia?

Conversely, when you are riddled with a disease, or experience consistent long term pain, when your thoughts and emotions are directed towards joy, empowerment, happiness, you will see symptoms decrease, and even completely go away.

A customer of mine who was seeing a pain specialist for long term issues of pain stemming from a car accident explained to me how she is almost always in pain and how it zaps her energy. I began talking about the mind body and was wondering if emotions tend to influence her pain and energy. She replied by telling me that when she speaks to a particular friend on the phone, someone she really likes and always makes her feel happy, her pain completely goes away.

Monitor your emotions throughout the day. Notice when you feel a negative emotion taking hold of you, such as the ones listed above. Ask yourself if the emotion is necessary and is the situation really what you perceive it to be.

You might need to take a step back, allow yourself the ability to respond and not to react. Is this emotion a recurrent theme in your life? Do you feel this way often? If so, this could be a major influence to fuel any type of ill health that you are experiencing, or may in the future. The first step is the realization, once the realization is made, dramatic changes often follow.

Now that we know some of the most dis-empowering emotions for one's health, so what are some of the empowering ones?

- Love

- Joy

- Happiness

- Gratitude

- Appreciation

- Forgiveness

Is there room in your life for more of these? Since what you focus on expands and you attract more of, we would have to guess the answer would be, YES! Imagine what your life would be like when you begin acting out of love, joy, happiness, gratitude, forgiveness and appreciation.

In section three we will speak about a gratitude list, and how focusing on this on a regular basis can literally reprogram your other emotions as well as what experiences you draw to yourself in life. You will learn how just by looking at things with gratitude you can increase your happiness by 25%.

When you act out of emotional react-ability, you tend to make choices that are not to your benefit. One thing that comes to mind that we see practically every day is binge eating, usually on "junk" food. Binge or "trance-eating" as we call it, generally has a powerful emotional attachment. With trance eating we are pacifying and avoiding the emotion in question. The problem is, the emotion does not go away and the trance eating only hurts us. This is no different than a drug which is prescribed that acts only as a bandage coving symptoms, avoiding getting to the root of the problem.

As we have outlined in this chapter, emotions are very powerful and they can have a direct effect on your health. In the resource section in the back you will find a description of tapping, or EFT, something which I find to be a very powerful and proven technique to take the fire out of negative emotions.

ACTIONS & HABITS

"To keep the body in good health is a duty...otherwise we shall not be able to keep our mind strong and clear" - **Buddha**

Up until now we have placed an enormous importance on the non-physical world, though we do not want to lose sight of the mass importance of the physical. Without taking empowering actions and developing empowering habits all the work that we do on our inner health will have no place to manifest and stick.

Through the manifestation of health, the real pinnacle of what we notice from day to day is our actions which lead to our habits. Our actions are physical. They are tangible.

They are the end result of a journey that began with past and present conditioning. They are also the beginning to the journey that lays ahead, the journey of creating new, empowering sources of conditioning.

Actions eventually become habits. Habits are what we regularly do or don't do. A habit can be a not-doing. Not finishing a task can be a habit. Not attending to a certain responsibility can be a habit. Habits essentially create who you are from the physical realm.

Actions and habits decide if you eat that food. Actions and habits decide if you smoke that cigarette. Actions and habits decide if you drink too much. Actions and habits decide if you think positive thoughts, control your emotions, and what reality you choose to create for yourself.

Where your inner health can affect your outer health, healthy actions and habits will make working on your inner health even easier. You may have heard the saying to "treat your body like a temple," and often people refer to this as eating right, getting plenty of rest, and exercise. Also remember, it's about love without judgment, forgiving yourself for unhealthy actions you might have taken and letting go of the past experiences which still bother you on some level today.

FORGIVENESS

"Forgiveness is the best thing you can do for your well-being"

-Consolee Nishimwe

Where speaking of forgiveness might not seem like it fits talking about the physical realm, forgiveness has a direct relationship to the actions and habits which mold our lives, especially the disempowering ones.

Forgiveness is looking at yourself and other people with the spiritual knowledge of their innocence rather than the mortal perception of guilt. There are so many physical actions and habits others may take and we may take against ourselves, that leaves us in a negative state, allowing the ego to dispense the negative self-talk which tends to recycle itself. Forgiveness surrenders the very aspect of mind that we think protects us from further hurt.

Forgiveness is strength, not a weakness. By forgiving we do not grant victory to those who wronged us, even if that is ourselves, instead we surrender the aspect of the mind that is blocking us to make our simple shifts in perception and healing. Not forgiving is granting ultimate power to our ego, allowing it to shape our reality, and this includes our health.

Chapter 7

Food

"Let thy food be thy medicine and thy medicine be thy food"

- Hippocrates

When we talk about food, what I really want to get across is not about good food and bad food; let's just talk about eating real food. So much food on the grocery store shelves is not food, this stuff is created in a factory, and it's highly processed, genetically modified and contains ingredients which are not natural ingredients in our food chain.

A healthy diet, by definition, means plenty of vegetables, fruits and varied protein sources such as eggs, fish, and a variety of meats. A healthy diet should be lean, clean, and free (or as free as possible) from the toxins of our modern food supply: pollutants, nitrites, growth hormones, antibiotics, genetically modified organisms, pesticides from feed and chemical sanitizers or irradiation used in processing.

Time and time again, research has pointed to the benefits of a Mediterranean diet, and these are no coincidences, much of the basis being a high healthy fat diet, which is contradictory to the American Heart Association low fat model.

Here's a great example comparing a Mediterranean based diet VS- the American Heart Association style diet. Published online by the *New England Journal of Medicine*, findings from the landmark Spanish PREDIMED (PREvención con DIeta MEDiterranea) trial report that a Mediterranean diet including nuts, primarily walnuts, reduced the risk of cardiovascular diseases (myocardial infarction, stroke or cardiovascular death) by 30 percent and specifically reduced the risk of stroke by 49 percent when compared to a reference diet consisting of advice on a low-fat diet (American Heart Association guidelines).

According to lead researcher Dr. Ramon Estruch, "the results of the PREDIMED trial are of utmost importance because they convincingly demonstrate that a high vegetable fat dietary pattern is superior to a low-fat diet for cardiovascular prevention."

The trial included 7,447 individuals (55 to 80 years old) at high cardiovascular risk who were followed for an average of 4.8 years. Participants in the study were randomized into one of three intervention diets: Low-fat diet (control group), Mediterranean diet supplemented with extra-virgin olive oil (50 ml per day), or a Mediterranean diet supplemented with 30 g mixed nuts, primarily walnuts, per day (15 g walnuts, 7.5 g almonds and 7.5 g hazelnuts.) Both the Mediterranean diet supplemented with nuts as well as the Mediterranean diet enriched with extra-virgin olive oil reduced the risk of cardiovascular diseases by 30 percent.

There are some major take a ways here. First and foremost, once again a low-fat diet is not what leads to a healthy heart; it's a high vegetable and high healthy fat diet. We have seen that when adding olive oil as well as the benefits of vegetarian based omega-3's in walnuts, a dramatic improvement in the cardiovascular outcomes.

Here are some general healthy eating and dieting tips:

- Whole Foods rich in phytonutrients

- Organic, GMO Free

- 8 to 10 servings of colorful vegetables and fruits every day- different colors, different beneficial attributes, phytonutrients and antioxidants.

- Healthy liquid choices; water, water with lemon, green tea, unsweetened tea, pomegranate juice.

- Healthy proteins and Lean animal protein- fish, turkey, chicken, buffalo, lean lamb, vegetables, nuts, beans, tofu

- Good oils- olive, sesame, nut oils, avocado

- Good fats- Omega 3 fatty acids, cold water wild salmon, sardines, herring, seaweed, coconut oil, avocado

- High fiber- whole beans, whole grains, nuts, seeds, vegetables

- Low in saturated fats- grass fed beef (less saturated fat)

- Good Carbohydrates- low glycemic, high fiber

- Limit or avoid dairy and wheat

GMO's

GMO's, or genetically modified organisms, should not be considered food; they are a science experiment which has gone terribly wrong leaving our environment and health in their wake.

The GMO debate keeps heating up and you will constantly hear two strongly opposing sides. Where a study comes out implicating GMO foods in an issue of health, other scientists will speak out in an attempt to discredit the study and the media takes it and runs with it.

You will soon see why I have begun recommending a GMO free diet to many of my clients. Food is very powerful, and as our food supplies have gradually shifted away from real foods, and more of a chemical composition, certain disease states have been skyrocketing.

For years we have seen stories implicate mammary tumors in mice, to organ failure in rats, and recently, how glyphosate induces breast cancer via estrogen receptors. Research has been implicating the health problems with GMO's for a very long time, although now it is finally being shared through the media on a large scale.

We have seen countries around the globe (with the exception of the US) begin to ban GMO crops, and other countries have begun saying, "thanks but no thanks" to our wheat exports due to the cross-contamination and genetic pollution problems with GMO's. This is a real problem.

The whole GMO issue centers on Roundup, the herbicide with the active ingredient known as glyphosate.

The seeds that Monsanto makes are genetically engineered to withstand the glyphosate while the weeds around them perish. In recent years we have found that organisms and weeds build a resistance to the glyphosate, requiring more and more to glyphosate be applied to the crops as well as adding other chemicals to the mixture, thus these chemicals are deposited into our food system at ever increasing amounts, making their way to the human body. Additionally, farmers have found the glyphosate being linked to an issue of sick soil, contributing to "super weeds", further leading to unhealthy crops and a major challenge to our environment and agriculture.

The Shikamate Pathway, The Gut, Your Health

Before we go further in talking about how it affects our health, I don't want you to fall into the belief trap that glyphosate is non-harmful to the human being as Monsanto has been preaching for many years. You might have heard Monsanto say that the human biology does not use the shikamate pathway, it is not in our cells, thus is harmless. Although falling in line with their bad science, this is untrue.

Glyphosate kills organisms by disrupting what is known as the shikamate pathway which is the biosynthetic sequence employed by plants and bacteria to generate the aromatic amino acids: phenylalanine, tyrosine, and tryptophan.

The good bacteria that is in your gut does in fact contain the shikamate pathway, and this is where GMO seeds as well as other food sources, lawns and gardens treated with glyphosate can be detrimental to your health- and all the more reason to avoid GMO's and supplement with probiotics daily.

As you know, the gut bacteria play many roles in our health, from aiding in digestion, to synthesizing vitamins, detoxifying xenobiotics, participating in immune system homeostasis and gastrointestinal tract permeability. And there are a lot of gut bacteria; they outnumber the cells in our body, 10:1, thus the argument that since our cells do not have a shikamate pathway, then glyphosate is safe, is ridiculous- let's look a bit deeper in how it affecting gut bacteria, it affects our whole health.

It is the result of the damage by glyphosate to the shikamate pathway to the good bacteria in our guts that links GMO foods to most of the diseases associated with the western diet; gastrointestinal disorders, diabetes, heart disease, depression, autism, cancer, Alzheimer's disease and others.

By disrupting the beneficial bacteria which we rely on to crowd out the pathogens, pathogens then begin to over grow leading to an issue of dysbiosis. This leads to inflammation, which then leads to leaky gut, where toxins readily spill into the bloodstream and can even make their way to the brain.

This process opens the door for wide spread nutritional absorption issues which lead to deficiencies, and opens up the possibilities for inflammatory and auto-immune conditions as well as disease of detoxification.

Glyphosate plays many roles, although I think it is important to point out the two major issues it causes; (1) wide spread nutritional deficiencies, (2) toxicities in the body.

Nutritional Deficiencies

As mentioned above, the shikamate pathway leads to the creation of aromatic amino acids. If the gut bacteria are damaged from the glyphosate in foods, these amino acids (part of the building blocks of proteins) do not get created.

Some downstream deficiencies and affects cause by depletions of aromatic amino acids.

dl-phenylalanine

- dl-phenylalanine is a precursor to tyrosine, thus can lead to tyrosine deficiency.

- dl-phenylalanine is needed for the production of melanin, the skins natural sunscreen, thus could affect the bodies natural skin protection and influence rates of skin cancer.

- dl-phenylalanine is a precursor for dopamine, epinephrine and nor-epinephrine, thus can have wide implications in behavioral issues as well as how one responds to stress.

L-Tryptophan

- Tryptophan deficiency can lead to serotonin deficiency which can lead to behavioral issues such as increased anxiety, trouble sleeping, decreased mood, increased irritability, and increased irrationality.

- Tryptophan deficiency can lead to problems with appetite, weight gain and even obesity. People tend to stay hungry, have more hunger cravings, which can all affect and lead to issues of obesity.

- There have been numerous reported incidences of when children who have behavioral issues go on a GMO free diet, how aggressiveness declines and other issues improve within days to weeks of the diet.

L-Tyrosine

- Decreased tyrosine can lead to decreased dopamine levels which can have a direct effect on Parkinson's disease.

- Tyrosine is one of the two ingredients to levothyroxine (T4) - along with iodine, thus can lead to decreased thyroid production.

Sulfur

Sulfur and sulfite play many roles in healthy methylation. Deficiencies can lead to:

- Impaired glucose metabolism since due to the lack of sulfur/sulfite. The cells have an impaired ability to store the sugar in the cells, and sugar builds up in the blood stream, ushering in hyper-insulinemia, pre-diabetes, weight gain and more.

- Imbalanced production of downstream amino acids such as methionine and cysteine leading to a rise in homocysteine, a risk factor for cardiovascular and Alzheimer's disease.

- Wide spread nutritional deficiencies due to impaired absorption via leaky gut. With a sulfur deficiency, the cells in the intestinal track become loose, and gaps appear which can lead to a loss of nutrients. This can be prevalent in those with digestive issues such as IBS, reflux, ulcers, which can lead into auto-immune conditions such as Crohns disease. It is important to note that there are numerous reported cases of individuals who have had digestive disturbances, from simple reflux, to IBS and others who have been recommended to go on a GMO free diet, to have symptoms improve dramatically in as little as days to weeks.

eNOS (endothelial nitrous oxide)

- Glyphosphate has shown to block the production of eNOS, which is endothelial nitrous oxide. Deficiencies of eNOS have shown to lead to cardiovascular complications such as elevated blood pressure.

- Additionally, eNOS helps produce sulfate, thus further leading to complications caused by sulfate deficiencies.

Nutrients such as Calcium, Magnesium, Iron and Cobalt

Broad deficiencies have been linked to GMO's having a wide array of effects such as leading to illness due to lack of nutritional relevancy, to over-eating to prevent starvation, just to get an adequate amount of nutrition, albeit contained in the delivery of more and more calories.

Cobalt deficiency has led to a deficiency in cobalamin, which plays a very important role in inflammation of the myelin sheath which protects nerve endings. This has known implications such as paralysis due to the inflammation of the spinal cord, neurological symptoms, Multiple Sclerosis, issues of detoxification, autism, etc. Throughout this book you will be learning about the importance of other minerals as well, thus highlighting the gravity of such deficiencies from GMO's.

Toxicities

Many of the major diseases of today have an environmental element and impaired detoxification associated to them. Autism would be a perfect example, and while most research and reporting is directed towards a genetic linkage, much more must be done to look at the environmental factors.

When I say environmental, this is inside and out, what goes on inside the body, and what is around the body which influences it.

Toxic Phenols

When the gut bacteria are not able to make the amino acids mentioned above, what they do end up creating are toxic phenols instead. Toxic phenols have been implicated in many disease states, as well as challenging the detoxification capacity of the body. They have shown to lead to or influence inflammation of the liver, hepatitis, and even liver cancer.

Ammonia

Ammonia is a gas which travels easily throughout the body. Ammonia has been implicated in issues of encephalopathy, as well as in Alzheimer's disease. Where there are some gut bacteria which can actually breakdown glyphosate, the end result is an increased production of Ammonia.

Formaldehyde

Depending on someones diet, this can be a kiss of death with GMO's. The artificial sweetener aspartame breaks down into formaldehyde, and so does certain GMO's. Roundup Ready Corn has shown to have upwards of 200 parts per million of formaldehyde. The permissible limit as outline by OSHA is somewhere between 0.75 ppm and 2 ppm. Formaldehyde can lead to destruction of DNA which supports the growth of cancer.

Blocks Cytochrome P450 Enzymes (CYP)

- The CYP system is designed to detoxify toxins in the liver including xenobiotics, drugs, toxic chemicals, endogenous and exogenous hormones and more.

- CYP plays an important role in cholesterol homeostasis, creations of bile acids, activation of Vitamin D, and blocks aromatase which plays a role in the metabolism and conversion of hormones. It is interesting to note that aromatase is often deficient in autistic children, a disease of environmental and impaired detoxification.

- With the role it plays in homeostasis of cholesterol, in addition to the plethora of cholesterol lowering drugs and activity, one must understand that cholesterol plays a very important role in brain health where it protects the cells from ion leaks and is important for synaptic transport. This basically can lead to the metabolic challenge of energy deficiency, as well as the promotion of type III diabetes (aka Alzheimer's disease.)

If you are dealing with any state of disease, I encourage you to navigate towards a GMO free organic diet for 4 to 8 weeks. See for yourself, and you might experience what many others have; significant resolution of symptoms and disease where you incorporate GMO free to your long term daily lifestyle.

Allergies and Food Intolerances

Food allergies and food intolerances are a major factor and often the big monkey wrench when it comes to someone's health. Food allergies and food intolerances can be developed towards any food, whether if it is a natural and organic whole food, or if it is processed, genetically modified, or filled with artificial colorings, preservatives, and sweeteners. A food allergy or intolerance happens when someone consumes food, the immune system reacts to it in an inflammatory response to what it considers to be a foreign/toxic agent.

There are some differences between food allergy and food intolerance. Food allergies account for approximately 5% of food reactions, happen immediately or within hours of consuming the food, and can be severe such as a rash, or an anaphylactic reaction such as fainting or where someone might have difficulty breathing. When being tested, food allergies are IgE immune mediated.

Food intolerances are more common accounting for about 95% of food reactions, they are more difficult to identify since they can happen within a few hours to a few days from consuming the food, and the symptoms are more subtle and can present themselves in many ways from skin rashes, eczema, difficulty sleeping, anxiety, behavioral difficulties and more. When being tested, food intolerances are IgG immune mediated.

As you will see, both food allergies and food intolerances make a very big impact on our health care system:

- 60% of US population has some sort of food response.
- $500 million a year is spent to treat food allergies and intolerances.
- From 1997-2007 there was a 185% increase in food reactions.
- From 1997-2002 there was a doubling of peanut allergies.
- 1/17 children under 3 year olds have some sort of food allergy/intolerance.
- There has been a 265% increase in hospital treatments and admittances.

There are numerous symptoms that are often not linked to food reactions, often resulting in unnecessary doctors' visits, testing, procedures and medications including:

- Anal itching
- Congestion, runny nose
- Anaphylactic, difficulty breathing
- Anemia
- Anxiety and Stress Disorders
- Digestive issues- pain, gas, diarrhea, constipation etc.
- Dark circles under eyes
- Eczema and other skin reactions
- Emotional outbursts
- Wrinkles under eyes
- Red earlobes
- Red eyes
- Ringing in the ears
- Restless, Irritability, agitation
- Restless leg syndrome
- Tension headaches
- Muscle cramps
- Decrease concentration and memory
- Increased ear wax
- Food addictions or cravings

In addition to direct symptoms caused by food reactions, there are many disease states which can further be aggravated by food allergies and intolerances including:

- Asthma

- Acne

- Auto-Immune

- Alzheimer's

- Cancer

- Cardiovascular

- Arthritis

- Neurological- ADD, ADHD, Autism

- Upper Respiratory Infections- chronic and recurring

- Ear infections- chronic and recurring

- Depression

- Menstrual irregularities

- Skin conditions such as eczema

- Insomnia

- Gastro Intestinal conditions including irritable bowel syndrome (IBS), Crohn's Disease and others

- Obesity

As the statistics shown above, food allergies and intolerances are on a dramatic rise, thus one would have to ask why. Often times it is due to the increased factory farming, industrialization of our food sources and ever growing problems with our foods being created in labs, the major increase we have seen in genetically engineered proteins and foods (aka GMO'-s) as well as they heavy use of antibiotics and growth hormones used in cows and other food producing animals.

We will be addressing the topic of vaccines a little later, although it is interesting to point out that the sharp rise of peanut allergies is being linked to the excipient ingredients in vaccines. In the book *The Doctor Within*, it is suggested that vaccines may be largely responsible for both the advent and increased prevalence of peanut allergy, noting that many vaccines and even antibiotic drugs contain, or were made using, excipients potentially derived from peanut oil. Since it is a relatively inexpensive oil to produce, refined peanut oil apparently became widely adopted as an excipient of choice in the production of vaccines during the 1960s, according to some reports, and peanut-derived excipients are still believed to be in use today for this purpose.

If you feel that you might be experiencing a particular food allergy or intolerance, here are some of the most common foods (and non-foods) to cause reactions.

Common Food Allergens/Intolerances

- Eggs
- Milk
- Peanuts
- Tree nuts
- Soy
- Wheat
- Fish
- Shell fish
- Chocolate
- Citrus fruits
- Coffee
- Corn
- Dairy

- Food additives
- Pesticide residue
- Refined Sugar
- Tomatoes
- Yeast
- Gluten and Gliaden
- Food additives
- Pesticide residues
- Genetically Engineered Foods

There are a number of different ways to be tested for food reactions. The important thing to understand is that there are differences between allergies and intolerances and how your body responds. As mentioned above, a food allergy is IgE immune mediated and intolerance is IgG mediated. So, if a doctor is only checking via IgE, then intolerances which are much more common can be missed.

Excitoxins

Excitotoxins are substances added to foods and beverages that literally stimulate neurons to death causing brain damage, mitochondrial damage, genetic mutations and other problems of varying degrees. Excitotoxins found in foods are usually ingredients such as MSG and aspartame. Basically a cell will become over-excited ultimately leading to cell damage and death.

There are numerous illnesses attributed to excitotoxity, often labeled as 'mysterious,' not being recognized as part of the problem including; promote growth and spread of cancer, sudden cardiac death, increased carbohydrate cravings (MSG), metabolic syndrome and leptin insensitivity, dementia and brain atrophy, seizures, autoimmune disorders, migraine headaches, obesity, diabetes, neurodegeneration disorders (Alzheimer's, Autism, ALS, Parkinson's, Huntingdon's), ADD, allergies, asthma, arthritis, celiac disease, chronic fatigue syndrome, colitis, crohn's disease, depression, epilepsy and seizure disorders, fibromyalgia, hypertension, thyroid disorders, infertility, insomnia, and many others.

One of the big problems with MSG is that it not only is it so prevalent in our foods, it can be elusively disguised in our foods. The following is a list of different names and ingredients where MSG can be found or described; MSG, gelatin, monosodium glutamate, monopotassium glutamate, autolyzed plant protein, natural flavors, hydrolyzed Vegetable Protein, hydrolyzed milk protein, autolyzed Yeast, natural beef flavoring, kombu extract, bouillon, natural pork flavoring, barley malt, natural chicken flavoring, RL-50, broth, natural seasonings, textured protein, calcium caseinate, sodium caseinate, glutacyl, malt extract, hydrolyzed oat flour, tamari, malt flavoring, hydrolyzed plant protein, zest and others.

Some of the big areas where aspartame is found are in sauces, flavorings and spices, broths, baby food, vegan and soy products, food bars, malt extracts, flavored syrups for coffees, protein bars and drinks, and beverages.

Common areas where aspartame is found are in sugar free colas and drinks, cereals, medications, breath mints, gum, hard candy, flavored syrups, iced tea, ice cream, instant cocoa, pudding, nutrition bars and protein shakes, packaged diet foods and shakes, and yogurt.

One of the more recent disturbing events has come from the dairy industry. When we talk about osteoporosis you will hear my feelings on milk and dairy in regards to bone health where it has not been shown to prevent bone fractures and some studies have shown it can increase them. In addition to this, approximately ¾ of the world population is genetically intolerant to dairy. Milk is full of saturated fat, thus increasing its cardiovascular risks, and if it is not organic, it is full of antibiotics and growth hormones.

And now The International Dairy Foods Association (IDFA) and the National Milk Producers Federation (NMPF) have filed a petition with the FDA requesting the agency "amend the standard of identity" for milk and 17 other dairy products. Amend the identity??? How far do they want to separate us from real food?

This was done to provide for the use of any "safe and suitable" sweetener as an optional ingredient — including non-nutritive sweeteners such as aspartame to deceive you by not having a strong indication of its usage on the label.

So, as you can see, the food industry is going to all levels to fill our foods with flavor enhancing and arguably addictive foods which might have some major implications on one's health.

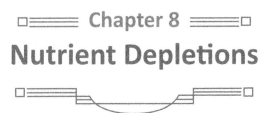

Chapter 8

Nutrient Depletions

When we start looking at therapy to reduce or mitigate someone's symptoms or risk factors to a disease, we cannot continue to overlook nutrient depletions. As you will see, nutrient depletions are due to many reasons; diet, age, lifestyle, quality of foods, and medications.

Often times if someone is dealing with a symptom or risk factor of a disease, in one way or another they are already dealing with some sort of nutrient depletion. Then, if a medication is added to the mix, we are looking at either making current depletions worse, or adding a host of others-all the while the body is screaming for some holes to be plugged.

Nutritional Depletion's are one of the most over-looked and ignored realities that are crippling our Nation's health and can play a role in every disease. Aside from extreme deficiencies and malnutrition leading to disease states such as beriberi, visible goiters, scurvy and others; many nutritional deficiencies go unnoticed leading to everything from problems with your heart, difficulty sleeping, lack of energy, difficulty losing weight, and more.

Because much of this is not taught in Medical and Pharmacy schools, people's health often flies under the radar and falls victim to problems and disorders that can possibly be very easily treated, and even prevented.

There are four main factors to nutritional deficiency:

1. Diet

2. Lifestyle

3. Age

4. Prescription and non-prescription medications

Have you ever gone to the doctor, maybe complaining of depression, low energy, difficulty sleeping, and after all tests are run…everyone is just scratching their heads?

…Or worse yet you are told it's all in your head?

When the body is depleted of vitamins, minerals, enzymes and amino acids, it weakens, making it susceptible to a whole host of diseases, malfunctions and overall loss of wellbeing.

In fact, researchers in the Journal of the American Medical Association stated,

> *"Suboptimal vitamin states are associated with many chronic diseases including cardiovascular disease, cancer, and osteoporosis. It is important for physician's to identify patients with poor nutrition or other reasons for increased vitamin needs."*

The Journal continues,

"Most people do not consume an optimal amount of all vitamins by diet alone...it appears prudent for all adults to take vitamin supplements."

Diet

Reasons for nutritional depletions in diet include; soil which is depleted and not replenished with important minerals such as zinc and magnesium, fruits and vegetables begin to lose their nutrient value immediately after being picked (Example-storing asparagus for one week can cause it to lose up to 90 percent of its vitamin C), the longer you cook fruits and vegetables- the fewer nutrients remain, processing, blanching, sterilizing, canning, and freezing foods all decrease the foods nutritional value, and certain limited dietary practices themselves can lead to a host of depletions, such as extreme high protein and low carbohydrate diets, and even an unbalanced vegetarian diet.

Age

Nutritional deficiencies due to aging are also very common. As you age, your body begins to produce less of its own nutrients such as; Vitamin D, Glutathione, Alpha-lipoic Acid, CoEnzyme Q10, and others; thus requiring the body to search for such nutrients elsewhere. By not supplementing with external sources coupled with deficiencies caused by other factors - could we be accelerating the disease and aging process?

Lifestyle

Lifestyle nutritional deficiencies are also a big deal. There are many aspects to our lifestyle that can affect our nutritional status; risk factors such as: stress, consuming alcohol, smoking, environmental challenges, inside the home and out.

Now that we see what nutritional depletions can come just from everyday living, let's talk about what many consider to be the straw that can break the camel's back- drug induced nutrient depletions.

Medications

Many people do not realize that almost all medications will cause drug induced nutrient depletions, aggravating or even being a route cause for many states of disease. The printouts you get with your prescriptions will talk about side-effects, although the fact is many of these side-effects can also be attributed to drug induced nutrient depletions and it seems no one says a word.

As you have seen, there are various challenges against a healthy nutritional status, do not allow drug induced nutrient depletions to be "the straw that breaks the camels' back."

Here is a quick example. It is estimated that over 50% of North Americans are deficient in magnesium and don't even know that they are. Being deficient in magnesium can leave you twice as likely to die form a cardiovascular event.

Magnesium is responsible for a number of critical heart healthy actions to maximize heart health including: decreases blood vessel constriction, improves glucose uptake by insulin, improves muscle strength and endurance, relaxes electrical impulses and encourages calmness, maintains the normal rhythm of your heart, metabolizes fats and carbohydrates for energy production, and increases HDL (good) cholesterol.

There are numerous medications to treat various cardiovascular disorders from blood pressure to even congestive heart failure which will ultimately lead to a depletion of magnesium, putting the heart at further risk- and seldom is this mentioned at the doctor's office or pharmacy counter.

Later in this book we will be talking about Metabolic Syndrome, which is a culmination of disease states including diabetes, high blood pressure, and high cholesterol. Metabolic syndrome is a reason for many medications being dispensed.

It is not uncommon that you will see someone on a statin drug for cholesterol, a beta blocker for blood pressure and heart rate, and a diabetes medication such as a sulfonylurea or combination with metformin, and maybe even a diuretic.

From these four medications alone, one person can be experiencing a depletion in; Co Enzyme Q10, vitamin E, magnesium, vitamin B12, vitamin B6, vitamin B1, zinc, potassium, folic acid and calcium. Just looking at the cardiovascular benefits B vitamins, Co Enzyme Q10, magnesium, folic acid, potassium and vitamin E provide, what are we setting people up for?

People are running on empty, they feel like crap, and I have seen time and time again that reintroducing these nutrients through quality supplementation can make a tremendous difference not only in how they feel, but in their lab markers as well.

Let me give you one last example, because it's a pretty big deal considering how many estrogen prescriptions, including birth control pills are dispensed.

Oral estrogen medications include most oral contraceptives (birth control), hormone replacement medications such as Prempro®, Premarin®, Cenestin®, Estrace®(estradiol), and compounds with go by names such as Bi-Est and Tri-Est.

Oral estrogen therapy has shown to decrease many vitamins in the B Vitamin Family such as: Folic Acid, Vitamins B1, B2, B3, B6, and B12 in the body possibly leading to a host of problems such as anemia, increased risk for heart disease, depression, neuropathies, birth defects, cervical dysplasia, memory loss, muscle weakness, problems with the Skin, mucous membranes and eyes, difficulty sleeping, and overall tiredness or lethargy.

Oral estrogen therapy has shown to decrease calcium in the body, possibly leading to osteoporosis, problems with development of teeth, impaired blood clotting function, and a reduction in the ability for cholesterol to make sex hormones.

Oral estrogen therapy has shown to deplete powerful anti-oxidants such as Vitamin C and Vitamin E, possibly leading to an impaired immunity, poor wound healing, increased free radical attack, easy bruising, increased risk of cardiovascular disease, PMS (premenstrual syndrome) and macular degeneration.

Oral estrogen therapy has shown to deplete minerals, amino acids and micro nutrients such as magnesium, selenium, zinc and tyrosine possibly leading to cardiovascular problems, PMS, osteoporosis, muscle cramps, trouble sleeping, impaired immunity, increased free radical attack, impairment of thyroid function, slowed wound healing, sexual dysfunction and more.

Whether you are looking just to stay healthy or you are currently taking medications and looking to find balance in your health and eventually transition off of the medication merry-go-round, drug induced nutrient depletions is one of the first areas to be addressed.

For more information, check out *The Nutritional Cost of Drugs* by Jim LaValle RPh CCN, and Ross Pelton RPh CCN, or *Drug Muggers* by Suzy Cohen RPh.

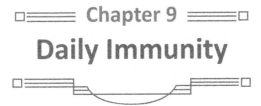

Chapter 9
Daily Immunity

Remember earlier when we spoke about transitioning from industrial age medicine to information aged medicine and how self-care should be the starting point and as someone transitions over to a health care practitioner for total care costs increase and one loses a bit of self-sufficiency? One of the areas that that I feel would benefit most is daily immunity; cough, colds, flu and even seasonal allergies- all areas that can advance into bigger problems of health if not attended to.

Even the CDC recognizes the problems that have developed from the over-prescribing of medications such as antibiotics and have begun a program urging practitioners to prescribe them only when clearly necessary. Whether it's that a patient feels like they got their money's worth and does not want to leave empty handed, or the doctor just wants to get them out of their office, the over-prescribing of antibiotics is leading to major problems such as drug resistant bacteria, known as super bugs.

These are strains of bacteria which have "evolved" in response to trying to stay alive every time an antibiotic is being thrown at them, and eventually become resistant, leaving people acquiring infections that mainstream medicine has run out of arsenal to fight it with. All the while preventative, or natural options would have done the trick. Additionally, it might be a virus where an antibiotic (against bacteria) serves no purpose, and might add insult to injury by weakening the immune system by destroying the immune supporting good bacteria in the digestive tracts.

So here are my 5 basic steps to staying healthy, any time of the year.

1. **Healthy diet**- For so many reasons we must navigate away from the standard American diet (S.A.D.) which can influence so many disease states- and one's general immunity is no different. White sugars, white flours, refined and processed foods, artificial flavorings, colorings and sweeteners can all take aim at ones immune system. Food intolerances can play a very big role here as well. Many issues can be related to foods such as dairy or even gluten. Countless times we have seen children what seemed to be maintenance antibiotics for ear infections, when a dairy intolerance could have been the causative factor.

2. **Stress reduction**- This is a common theme you will find in this book, and it is ever so important for daily health and wellness. One should not find it a coincidence that cough, cold and flu season hits high gear after the holiday season, after stress has been running high (along with not the healthiest foods being consumed) and people suddenly fall victim to every little cold and virus that comes their way.

3. **Optimized vitamin D3 therapy**- Vitamin D3 has so many benefits and it is important to optimize our doses. Optimized therapy would require testing ones active vitamin D blood levels and supplementing with vitamin D3 if levels are low, with a goal of between 40 and 60 ng/ml.

4. **Probiotics**- Probiotics are critical. The 'gut' or digestive tract is ground zero for our immune system. Probiotics, or 'good bacteria' in the digestive tract are often challenged by diet, medication therapy, stress and other issues of lifestyle – and to provide foundational immune support, probiotics are paramount. If you choose not to add a good probiotic on a regular basis, at least remember to do so with any antibiotic prescription you take…I generally recommend a 2 week supplementation of a quality, multi-strain probiotic after antibiotic therapy. Recolonizing good bacteria after antibiotic therapy is a huge area that constantly goes unaddressed by pharmacists and doctors throughout the country.

5. **Foundational nutrition via quality multi-vitamin**- A multivitamin is designed to "plug the holes" so to speak, and this has far reaching benefits on your health, wellness and immunity. Additionally there is plenty of research alluding to deficiency in certain nutrients such as zinc and selenium can lead to a higher chance of getting sick.

Years back we were researching the ins and outs of moving to Hawaii and maybe buying a coffee farm. We came across a master in the field of growing coffee organically and he said something in regards to how to avoid pesticides and herbicides. He said if you keep the host (the plant) strong and healthy, it should be able to fend off attack and not fall victim to bugs. I believe it is the exact same for the human body, and antibiotics and flu vaccines do not make the host stronger.

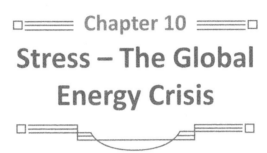

Chapter 10

Stress – The Global Energy Crisis

"Every stress leaves an indelible scar, and the organism pays for its survival after a stressful situation by becoming a little older."

\- Hans Selye

Our society is in an energy crisis; lack of energy, lack of focus, memory loss, weight gain, issues of libido, hormonal imbalances, and compromised immune systems are all symptoms that can be related to stress. When we talk about stress, it's all about how we manage it and adapt to it, or mismanage it and don't adapt to it, and how it plays out on our adrenal glands. The fact is, almost every known disease can be adversely affected by mismanaged, ignored or unrecognized stress, and few people are doing anything about it.

The Truth about Stress

Time and time again, science and medicine shows that stress kills, although all too often, people do not address the impact that stress can make on their health. Stress is a physiological reaction that people experience, stemming from emotional, physical and mental sources. The part of the body that is responsible for dealing with stress and providing us the hormones and natural body chemicals to do so are the adrenal glands. The adrenal glands sit in an area above the kidneys and are responsible for producing adrenal hormones such as cortisol, DHEA, and adrenaline.

The way we have been designed is to deal with stress in an adaptive way. Stress is supposed to come in spurts, we then alter our biochemistry (blood flow leaves organs such as the digestive tract and goes to muscles) to deal with and adapt- then it goes away and we go back to 'normal.'

We need stress, stress is part of our natural ability to grow, although the problem comes when stress is not managed such as now-a-days it seems stress never goes away, thus we are redefining a 'new normal'- and it's not a good one. When stress comes and goes or we learn to deal with it in a balanced fashion, it's a good thing, it's the unbalanced way we go about dealing with stress which affects our health negatively.

Scientist Hans Selye introduced the General Adaptation Syndrome model in 1936. In his work, Selye - 'the father of stress research', developed the theory that stress is a major cause of disease because chronic stress causes long-term chemical changes.

He observed that the body would respond to any external biological source of stress with a predictable biological pattern in an attempt to restore the body's internal homeostasis.

This initial hormonal reaction is your fight or flight stress response - and its purpose is for handling stress very quickly. The process of the body's struggle to maintain balance is what Selye termed, the *General Adaptation Syndrome.*

Pressures, tensions, and other stressors can greatly influence your normal metabolism. Selye determined that there is a limited supply of adaptive energy to deal with stress. That amount declines with continuous exposure.

Liking this to revving your car on high RPM's constantly without a rest; your engine will burn out at a faster rate. Your adrenal glands and your body are the same way. Your adrenal glands are asked to work over-time and this eventually leads to what has been termed Adrenal Fatigue. Adrenal Fatigue is when your adrenal glands have little left to give which in turn leads to the symptoms I mention below, as well as a depletion of other hormones (our body's messengers) throughout our system.

General Reasons for Stress

Often if you ask someone about stress in their life, they will not recognize or admit that it is making such a major impact on their health. Either they are conditioned to accept that stress is a constant, might make a joke about it to deflect the reality in a "who doesn't" sort of way, or they think that just because things do not seem stressful right now, that the stress from even years ago can't still me making a very big impact.

Below are some common, as well as some life-changing examples of stress that can have a major impact on one's health. And remember, just because a stress related incident or experience happened years ago, does not mean it cannot affect you today.

Over-committing - This is about spreading yourself too thin, over booking and taking on too many responsibilities. Not saying 'no' when you really need to say 'no.'

Over-Stimulation - Not finding time for 'time out'…recognizing the body needs rest and renewal and time away from excessive stimulation from the outside world. One must recognize the need for silence, quiet time, op-posed to all the background noise people live with to drown out the silence such as running TV's and radio's when often they are not consciously lis-tened to.

Over-Connected – Being a slave to modern day 'conveniences' and falling into electronic OCD, such as cell phones, email, social networking sites, etc. It is important to realize the benefits of 'disconnecting' and to find the time to disconnect on a regular basis.

Loss of a Loved One- Death is part of the natural balance of life, although it can be very traumatic and difficult to deal with and in many ways can have a long lasting impact if not dealt with. This is one of the problems I feel with the over-prescribing of anti-depressants and psychotropic medications; they do not allow us to learn and grow from our losses. This has been proven by the work and the writings of the Austrian neurologist and psychologist Viktor Frankl, MD.

Frankl taught that people can discover meaning and purpose in their lives in three ways: by doing work that matters, by loving others unconditionally, and by finding meaning in their suffering. All of us are guaranteed to experience loss and grief in our lives. But we can choose how to respond and react to that suffering. Frankls' experience on stress comes from his experience as a concentration camp inmate which led him to discover the importance of finding meaning in all forms of existence, even the most sordid ones, and thus have a reason to continue living.

Loss of Income- Becoming a bigger issue in this day and age, loss of income can challenge us financially, as well as ones confidence and self-image.

Loss of Health- Loss of health has an impact on all areas of life, finance, happiness, relationships, etc. As I mentioned in the introduction, life can throw a lot of challenges at us, and none will kill us…accept challenges to our health.

Loss of Location- Moving is recognized as one of the major and often unidentified sources of stress, especially when one leaves support structures behind. Having to make new friends, changing schools or jobs, even losing identity that one might gain from a geographical area can result in a major impact on one's life.

Below is a list of symptoms related to stress. Take a look at them; see how many of these symptoms affect you. And keep in mind, many symptoms can be related to other imbalances of health, such as low thyroid disease, thus important to look at the body in a holistic manner as well as understand that stress can have a compounding effect on other disease states as well.

Symptoms of Stress and Adrenal Fatigue

- Fatigue
- Nervousness
- Irritability
- Depression
- Frustration
- Apathy
- Vertigo or dizziness
- Weakness
- Cravings
- Headaches
- PMS (Premenstrual syndrome)
- GI Disruption/ Acid Reflux
- Constipation
- Irritable Bowel
- Anxiety
- Panic
- Decreased Memory
- Confusion
- Insomnia and/or trouble getting to sleep
- Indecisiveness
- Procrastination
- Avoidance
- Increased Drug and Alcohol Use
- Decreased self-worth

- Decreased spontaneity
- Decreased creativity
- Lowered Endurance
- Exercise intolerance
- Lack of zest, melancholy
- Weight gain/belly fat
- Decreased immunity
- Hypoglycemia (low blood sugar)
- Decreased appetite
- Chronic fatigue syndrome
- Impotence
- Infertility
- Decreased sexual interest
- Disorganized
- Heart races or pounds

Stress Is A Perception and Interpretation of Energy

Our perception of the stress without objectively interpreting it can be our worst enemy; this has proven to be an issue with most people. You might have a lot going on, many irons in the fire, that's just life. But, due to a faulty ability to look at how to handle stress objectively- stress at times can get the best of you.

The basis of stress and how it affects you is energy, and the quality of the energy. Keep in mind, you never really lack energy, energy is within all matter; although you could experience more negative energy than positive energy, or more low energy than high energy- it's the quality of energy that matters as we spoke about earlier in the works of Dr. Bruce Lipton.

What I would like to share with you next I learned from Tony Schwartz and Jim Loehr and their book, *The Power of Full Engagement*. Where this book is focused on an individual's high performance, I find it critical in today's culture in regards to health; I regularly share this with my clients and highly recommend it to you.

The feelings of being burned out, depressed, exhausted, hopeless and defeated are is low negative energy. Other emotions such as anger, fear, anxiety, defensiveness or even resentment are considered high negative energy.

When we properly manage the balance of stress and recovery, we should be feeling invigorated, confident, challenged, joyful, even connected which is high positive energy. Then in times of recovery we should feel relaxed, mellow, peaceful, tranquil and serene which is low positive energy.

Do any of these sound familiar? The goal is to live our lives in a state of positive energy balanced with the rhythmical changes of high and low.

Let's now talk about pulsating rhythms. Nature itself has a pulse, a rhythmic, wavelike movement between activity and rest. Think about the ebb and flow of the tides, the movement between seasons, and the daily rising of the sun. As human beings we are no different; our breathing, heart rates, brain waves, hormone levels, body temperature, and blood pressure are all guided by rhythmic balances.

It is the unnatural disconnect from our natural rhythmical tendencies and this is why as a society we are so stressed out which can often lead to issues of disease. You might have heard the term, 'being in your zone,' or 'being in state,' this I believe is the connection of our natural rhythmical tendencies and our individual values falling in line.

So what can we do about it? It's time to connect and disconnect.

As you go throughout your day, I suggest that you balance your times of focused work (being connected) with rebound time for relaxation (time to disconnect). For example, when you are at work or working on a project, go for 60 to 90 minutes of focused, uninterrupted work. Then take a 10 to 15 minute break to renew, and be strict with your time frames. It is important to note that during your times of work, not to multi-task, it is only inefficient, less productive and mind deadening. Also, during your time of rest and renewal, do not go to your television, computer, email or cell phone-you need to really disconnect from the electronic OCD that so many people experience.

Getting caught up in this electronic OCD cycle will hamper your body's ability to renew. Trying a breathing exercise, talking with an associate about something other than work, maybe sit and do nothing at all. Give this experiment a try and I am confident you will find yourself getting more done with more energy at the end of the day.

This energy crisis should hit close to home with much of our society, because stress and the actions that it takes on our bodies has implications with almost every disease, many which I listed previously.

The current allopathic medical system does little to recognize the reality of stress which our culture is in, which makes sense since it is not adequately taught in most schools of medicine and pharmacy.

In the current allopathic quick to prescribe model, someone might go to the doctor complaining of anxiety, stress, apathy, depression, maybe PMS (premenstrual syndrome), low libido, resistant weight loss, when in fact, all of these symptoms and disease states might have a major connection to stress.

Mismanaged and improper assessment of stress is a significant reason why countless prescriptions are overly and unnecessarily prescribed, while never getting to the real problem; from anti-depressants, to sleeping medications, synthetic hormones, and even pain relievers. These classes of medications lead to countless side-effects, drug interactions, and even deaths. All the while the medical system ignores what's really gone on, as well as the fact that stress can have deleterious effects on many other systems of the body; not just the adrenal glands leading to even more issues of health and disease.

In a holistic system of medicine we understand the impact that stress has on all areas of our health and our life and look to support the body from many different areas from lifestyle, to diet, mind-body medicine, supplements and proper hormonal balance. Proper assessment to understand exactly how stress is affecting one's health is critical, which the conventional medical system often ignores.

How do we turn the course or repair ourselves from adrenal burnout? We look at adrenal repair primarily as a threefold process; assess the reality, nutritional supplementation and relaxation techniques.

1. Recognize how someone is affected by stress, and how they function. Are they stressed and wired or stressed and tired. Is it affecting other areas of their health? Testing as shown below will help dial someone in targeting their needs, allowing us to know the degree of their adrenal imbalance and how it represents itself throughout the day.

2. Provide the appropriate vitamins and nutrients to feed the adrenal glands to begin the strengthening and rebuilding process, basically providing adrenal food. Implement herbal, adaptogenic, amino acid or even glandular support, which helps the body and adrenals to adapt to stress, allows the adrenals to kick back and relax so they do not overwork themselves while supporting levels of energy and stamina.

The nutrients responsible for the adrenal repair and rebuilding are full spectrum B Vitamins, Vitamin C and magnesium. Adaptogens are usually herbal preparations such as ashwagandha, ginseng, rhodiola and cordyceps. There are other supplements which can help with relaxation as well as help balance out adrenal hormones such as cortisol and DHEA. Amino acids and inhibitory neurotransmitters such as L-Theanine and GABA can further help with the cortisol levels, while at the same time promoting focus and calming a racing mind. Glandulars are actually tissue from the adrenal glands of animals, such as bovine, in which the body will recognize the protein involved to further support the strengthening and rebuilding process.

3. Relaxation techniques offer the perfect balance to nutritional supplementation. This would include meditation, breathing exercises, prayer, or even disciplines such as yoga, tai chi, and qigong. During our normal waking consciousness, the human brain emits what are called beta waves. As we settle into mediation, the brain shifts and begins to emit alpha waves and

sometimes even the deeper delta waves. Delta waves help us access the unconscious; reduce levels of cortisol, similar to the nutrients I mentioned. In fact, according to an article published by the American Public Health Association, people who practice Transcendental Meditation spend 11 percent less annually on health care than does the general population.

Testing For Adrenal Health

The gold standard for testing one's adrenal health and assess the effect it has over one's health is through saliva testing. A saliva test of both cortisol and DHEA allows the best assessment of the health of and how the adrenals are working, allowing someone to test optimally 4 times a day simply by spitting in a tube. Contrary, the conventional model would do a morning blood draw for cortisol, which would not give any value on how the adrenals are acting throughout the day.

Where this assessment gives a snap picture on what is happening today, what is even of more value is to have this test done on a regular basis, such as every year to gain assessment on trends. This would identify if ones cortisol levels are rising or dropping. If they are normal today, but were extremely high only a year ago, this could indicate adrenal output is seriously dropping, allowing the practitioner to act proactively to prevent a significant drop in activity.

Supplements for Stress

When recommending nutrients for stress, it is often not a one size fits all approach. It was mentioned earlier, that people can be at different areas of the continuum of stress. Some people might have high cortisol levels, others low. Some people might be stressed and tired while others are stressed and wired.

Below you will find a list of supplements based on category and how they influence the body. In any case I generally recommend getting on board with the foundational elements which as you will see are Vitamin C, B complex, and Magnesium. I also am a fan of some sort of adaptogen which further helps the body to adapt to stress, as well as supports what is known as the HPA (Hypothyroid, Pituitary, Adrenal) Axis, in which optimal communication between these glands supports optimal health. You will see adaptogens do have different qualities, where some might be more appropriate for someone than others.

Following is a list of some of the foundational nutrients, adaptogens, and ancillary supplements which have unique benefits and can help dial in an individual's needs. As always we recommend only the highest in quality supplements as well as to seek guidance in assessing your needs.

Foundational Nutrients to Feed Adrenals

- Vitamin C - optimal non corn source and in alkalinizing "buffered" product.

- B Complex - can purchase active b's such as Vitamin B6- p5p (pyridoxine 5 phosphate) opposed to pyridoxine. Belief is the body does not have to work hard to convert to active form. Active forms will also be in much lower strengths.

- Magnesium - High absorption forms include glycinate, citrate, orotate and aspartate. Common over the counter magnesium examples which are low in bioavailability, thus not in favor, are magnesium chloride and magnesium oxide.

Herbal Adaptogens (help the body to adapt to stress; support, feed and rebuild adrenal action, and provide energy)

- Cordyceps - Adrenal support, immune support, increases oxygen utilization, kidney support, antioxidant support, sexual enhancement, improves stamina and endurance.

- Ashwanganda - Adrenal support, immune support, anti-inflammatory action, antioxidant support, supports endurance and strength, often found in 'calming' adaptogenic adrenal support products.

- Ginseng - American more calming, Asian more stimulatory. Adrenal support, increases energy, antioxidant support, immune support, can support elevated blood sugar and insulin levels.

- Rhodiola - Adrenal support, supports endurance and strength.

- Relora - Combination of phellendedrom and magnolia extract. Has common support and adaptogenic to both cortisol and DHEA. (If too high, can bring it down, if too low, can help bring back up.) Has also shown benefits in stress related food cravings and effects on blood sugar.

   Amino-Acids/Inhibitory neurotransmitters (for focus and concentration and to calm an over-active mind, and promote relaxation)

- L-Theanine- Promotes brain alpha activity, focus and concentration.

- GABA- Inhibitory neurotransmitter, supports relaxation. Promotes brain alpha activity with some research showing it can suppress beta activity, and supports immune system.

- Glycine- Inhibitory neurotransmitter, supports relaxation.

Miscellaneous

- Phosphatidylserine (adaptive for stress, decrease cortisol levels, can elevate mood, support memory, focus and attention)

- Licorice (for energy and adaptive support- avoid in cases of high blood pressure, panic and anxiety)

- Adrenal Glandular's- Adrenal extracts are used to support the proper functioning of the adrenal glands, and are often used to reduce fatigue and moderate stress. When using glandular extracts, we recommend using only freeze dried, vacuum dried extracts which are sourced from pasture fed, pesticide-free bovine herds.

Adrenal Support Checklist

1. Testing. Optimally you will have a salivary adrenal test consisting of testing DHEA and Cortisol four times throughout the day. This will provide a snap shot of how your adrenals are working.

2. Diet. Refer to the chapter 7 for the backbone of a healthy diet, and when speaking of adrenals it is important to limit the amount of refined foods, sugars, flours and caffeine laden foods.

3. **Relaxation Techniques.** This plays an enormous role in ones adrenal health and overall wellbeing. Incorporating regular relaxation techniques and stress relieving strategies is a must. Refer to Part III, where I cover tools such as meditation, emotional freedom technique (EFT), and others.

4. **Supplements.** Incorporating a combination of foundational nutrition as well as other supportive supplements can serve someone very well. Often times the addition of other supplements such as adaptogens, the amino acids or even glandular's mentioned above can be of benefit. Depending on someone's needs, which can be dialed in by an experienced practitioner, will determine which supplements are appropriate.

Here are a few examples of products I recommend and why.

- If someone is stressed and tired, with no problems of high blood pressure or anxiety, I will often recommend a combination product with adrenal adaptogens, licorice and adrenal glandular's, such as ADR from Pure Encapsulations.

- If someone is stressed and tired, with problems of high blood pressure or anxiety, I will recommend a combination adaptogen product such as AdreneVive by OthoMolecular or Cortisol Calm from Pure Encapsulations. Cortisol Calm offers the benefits of L-Theanine and magnolia for additional cortisol support, along with the adaptogens rhodiola and ashwagandha. L-Theanine also provides additional support for focus and concentration.

- If someone is stressed and wired, and/or has problems with high blood pressure or anxiety, I will avoid licorice and adrenal glandulars.

5. **Exercise** - Exercise plays a very big role in healthy adrenal activity as well. The important thing is to dial in the appropriate exercise routine for your needs. For instance, if you are experiencing severe adrenal fatigue, then excessive exercise can be insult to injury.

See also: Sleep, Thyroid, Hormonal Health, Metabolic Issues, and Diet.

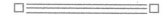

Chapter 11

Sleep

In my daily practice I see three types of sleepers. 1) Those that sleep heavy, are numb to their surroundings, and can sleep ten hours if you let them. With the exception of growing teenagers, adults who fit this profile in many cases are people who are at the far end of adrenal fatigue, the ones whose adrenals have been taking a beating for some time, and often their saliva cortisol tests will show a flat line. 2) Another group is those who either have trouble getting to sleep or wake up in the middle of the night, often with difficulty getting back to sleep. 3) The third group is the minority, the good sleepers. These are the people who get to sleep without a problem, sleep sound throughout the night and wake-up vibrant and excited to start the day. This third group is the goal for the other two.

Inadequate sleep has been linked to increase risk for diabetes, stroke, weight gain, impaired immune system, memory loss, and a recent report has tied regular good night's rest with living a long and healthier life. This requirement of sleep for a long and healthy life is alarming since it is reported that only 38% of Baby Boomer's actually get a consistent, good night's rest. This is a stark contrast to another survey of centenarians, a group of people living long healthy lives past 100 years old, and 71% say they get eight hours or more of sleep each night. This reason alone might be why it has recently been reported that members of the Baby Boomer generation are in significantly worse health than their parents were at the same age, according to a new study.

Reasons for not sleeping well can be linked to diet and lifestyle, hormonal imbalance's, drugs (prescription and recreational), "too connected" and over-stimulated by computers, TV's, cellphones, excessive alcohol and caffeine consumption, and or course…stress.

There are prescription agents that can get you sleeping, although they can be habit forming and many can actually suppress the body's production of melatonin, thus not an optimal long term solution. There over the counter drugs like Benadryl (diphenhydramine) found in many night time supplements, although people often wake-up groggy and these drugs have been implicated to impair mental cognition and memory.

Recently U.S. Food and Drug Administration (FDA) announced it is requiring the manufacturers of Ambien, Ambien CR, Edluar and Zolpimist, widely used sleep drugs that contain the active ingredient zolpidem, to lower current recommended doses. New data show that zolpidem blood levels in some patients may be high enough the morning after use to impair activities that require alertness, including driving. You might have heard of numerous other reports of increased sleep walking and other dangerous activities linked to these medications as well.

What are the natural alternatives? First, let's look at some lifestyle options. Try to get digestion out of the way before going to bed, finish your last big meal of the day at least three hours before bedtime. Avoid excessive carbohydrates and alcohol at nighttime, the increased sugar load can spike cortisol levels leaving you wide-awake in the early morning hours. Reduce stimulatory devices such as television, cellphones and computers too close to bedtime. It's ok to disconnect from modern technology, in fact it's good for you.

Since stress is a driver in almost all cases of trouble sleeping, it is imperative we look at lifestyle adaptors including relaxation techniques such as meditation, prayer and breathing exercises. I mentioned earlier about meditation and how it affects our brain waves.

I like to break it down into beta waves and alpha waves. Does your mind ever run out of control? Racing fast forward, bouncing back and forth, lack of focus and you just cannot calm it down? This is when our beta waves are running too high and/or alpha waves too low.

As we settle into mediation and a relaxed state, the brain shifts and begins to emit alpha waves which help balance out the excessive beta wave stimulation. I think it is imperative that we begin with such relaxation techniques, although let's see how nutritional supplementation can help.

As far as supplements, for simplicity I like to group them into five categories:

1. Melatonin- Melatonin, which is actually a hormone that decreases in production as we get older, helps to "reset" our time clock. Melatonin is also a powerful antioxidant. More is not always better with melatonin. A smaller dose might be just what someone needs, when a larger dose could cause them to have an unsettled sleep. Melatonin levels can be ordered and read by your physician for optimal wellness.

2. Natural, herbal central nervous system relaxants- Natural, herbal central nervous system relaxants including chamomile, valerian root, hops, lemon balm, passion flower and Seditol® (ziphisus and magnolia). A small percentage of people who take valerian root might experience an opposite effect, an unsettled sleep; people who experience hay fever could have a reaction to chamomile; and hops actually has estrogenic activity, thus might not be recommended in people with estrogen stimulated disease states such as prostate or breast cancer.

Seditol, a trade name with the active ingredient being ziphisus and magnolia, is one of my favorites in this category since it has been shown to support a restful sleep, has been reported to enhance daytime energy levels and to provide weight management support.

3. **Amino acids and inhibitory neurotransmitters-** Remember the brain wave thing? L-Theanine is an amino acid which promotes brain alpha waves supporting focus and concentration and calms a racing mind. GABA and Glycine are considered inhibitory neurotransmitters where they help to promote further relaxation. You can also see a reduction of cortisol levels with all of these, critical in an over-stressed society. The three of these work great for sleep, as well as daytime use for the 'stressed and wired', needing the calming benefits and help with focus, and concentration.

4. **Serotonin synthesis precursors-** 5HTP and L-Tryptophan have found their place in promoting emotional well-being as well as a restful sleep. As mentioned, these supplements are precursors to serotonin which is an important neurotransmitter involved in the regulation of brain activity responsible for emotion, appetite and sleep/wake cycles.

5-HTP is actually the intermediate in the synthesis of L-Tryptophan to serotonin. If one was to choose L-Tryptophan it is recommended to supplement with both Vitamin B6 and niacinamide, since these vitamins are needed for the conversion. Supplementation with 5-HTP will avoid this need. Both of these supplements have shown to promote relaxation as well as support healthy sleep quality, onset and duration. Due to both 5-HTP and L-Tryptophan's' ability to support serotonin levels, they are not recommended to be taking along with other medications such as antidepressants which stimulate increased levels of serotonin.

5. **Homeopathics/Flower Essences -** I find that both homeopathics and flower essences play a very effective role in supporting measures of sleep. Where they are different in how they are made, they have some similarities in low chance of interactions and side-effects with medications or herbals, and can be appropriate with almost any age group.

Sleep Checklist

1. **Relaxation Techniques.** This plays an enormous role in issues of sleep and overall wellbeing. Incorporating regular relaxation techniques and stress relieving strategies is a must. Refer to Part III, where I cover tools such as meditation, emotional freedom technique (EFT), and others. It is also important to recognize the stimulation that electronics and can have, such as watching TV, the computer and cell phones can have, thus leading to problems sleeping.

2. **Diet.** Refer to the chapter 7 for the backbone of a healthy diet, and when speaking of sleep it is important to limit the amount of refined foods, sugars, flours and caffeine laden foods.

3. **Exercise** - Exercise plays a very big role in sleep as it does with adrenals. The important thing is to dial in the appropriate exercise routine for your needs. For instance, if you are experiencing severe adrenal fatigue, then excessive exercise can be insult to injury. Exercising too close to bedtime can further cause issues with sleep.

4. **Supplements.** With sleep there are combination supplements which cast a wide net, or targeted supplements based on needs as we discussed above. I often find that people either have trouble getting to sleep, difficulty staying asleep (often waking up about 3 am), or both.

   Some of my favorite supplements are listed below, and serve as examples on how one can go about finding options which will work best for them. I often will begin with the recommendation of the GUNA-SLEEP, and then if needed add the Pure Tranquility to that if need some extra help, or still battle with issues of a racing mind. There are numerous products on the market; these are just a few of the ones I have found useful with my clients in my practice.

   GUNA-SLEEP- Homeopathic sleep aid which I have had great results with, works on wide range of sleep issues. Being a homeopathic, this is a good option to take when on other supplements or medications.

Pure Tranquility Liquid - Combination of L-theanine, GABA, and glycine. This works well to promote relaxation, calm a racing mind, and can even be used if someone wakes up in the middle of the night to get back to sleep.

Best Rest Formula - Multiple ingredient nutritional product, thus casts a wide net on issues of sleep; includes melatonin, 5 HTP, GABA, L-theanine, and an array of relaxant herbals.

See also: Adrenal, Thyroid, and Hormonal Health.

Chapter 12

What You Need To Know About Hormones

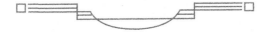

Hormonal Replacement Therapy (HRT) has changed dramatically over the past 10 to 20 years, and is probably one of the biggest improvements in integrative and longevity medicine. Pharmaceutical companies have been creating synthetic and non-human derived hormone medications for decades. Due to an increasing demand for what is known as Bio Identical Hormone Replacement Therapy (BHRT) there has been a swing towards customizes dosages with hormones which are identical to the ones the body naturally creates. Makes sense, right?

The artificial hormone chemicals that are created by drug companies are similar enough to exert an effect on the hormonal receptor, but different enough to produce different results, as well as come with their own bag of side-effects. This is where we find the true benefit of bio-identical hormones with nutritional support.

Hormonal balance is not a one-size fits all approach and what works for one person might not work for another. In our quest to provide hormonal soundness and balance, you will find that nutritional soundness is a key as well, and often begins with a previous topic of stress and adrenal health as we addressed previously. Aside from foundational nutrition, there are nutrients that can support both hormone application and metabolism in one's body, synthetic or natural.

Due to many issues of today; ever increasing stress, increasing toxins in our environment, and food sources that are drastically lacking nutritional relevancy soaked in pesticides and artificial hormones, and on top of that being genetically modified - our hormonal systems are going through hormonal exhaustion while at the same time being confused by medications and environmental toxins mimicking, but not matching, what our hormones should be doing.

Everyday more men and women are entering what is called Menopause for Women and Andropause for Men. In both cases there are physical and emotional issues related to a decline in the production of one's hormones.

Before we continue, I will be using the terms synthetic hormones and bio-identical or natural hormones. Bio-identical or natural hormones are hormones that are identical to the hormones that the natural body creates. Synthetic will refer to non-bio-identical hormones, as well as horse derived hormones used in a drug called Premarin ® (I wanted to make this point clear, because where the estrogen in Premarin is not bio-identical to a human; it can be called bio-identical to a horse.) I would also like to mention, just because its bio-identical does not mean that it cannot come without problems. Hormonal restoration therapy should only be done under proper testing and customization of doses for the needs of the patient.

Symptoms of Hormonal Imbalance and Beyond

Hormonal imbalance can mean different things for different people. I first want you to understand, it goes beyond the symptoms. Balanced hormones have shown to reduce risk factors to many diseases including dementia, heart disease, osteoporosis, and even cancer, regardless of the presence of symptoms. Where men and women both experience hormonal changes and often suffer imbalances, the experience can be different for everyone.

Many times people may not even realize that the symptoms they are experiencing are even hormonally related, or even that an illness they are suffering from has its hormonal roots. Where below I offer symptoms related to what is known as menopause (for women) and andropause (for men), that does not mean that you have to be 'at that time in life' to experience such symptoms. Decreasing hormones are becoming more common at earlier ages; it's the progressive exhaustion of the hormones we seek to balance for our health, happiness and overall wellbeing.

Where the definition of menopause is when there is no menstrual cycle for 12 consecutive months, there are many symptoms involved related to the time of peri-menopause to menopause. Here are a few of them, and as you can see, they play multiple roles and have multiple effects.

- Hot flashes
- Night sweats
- Vaginal dryness
- Mood swings
- Irritability
- Insomnia
- Depression
- Loss of sexual Interest
- Panic attacks
- Painful intercourse

- Osteoporosis
- Aching ankles, knees, wrists, shoulders, heels
- Weight loss
- Palpitations
- Varicose veins
- Urinary leakage
- Memory lapses
- Frequent urination

Where Andropause is not as concrete to diagnose as Menopause (menopause = no menstrual cycle for 12 consecutive months), there are many symptoms that follow along with the decline of male hormones such as:

- Decreased energy
- Decreased mental quickness
- Decreased desire for physical activity
- Decreased or loss of sexual interest
- Decreased muscle tone
- Increase in body fat especially in the mid-section
- Night sweats
- Trouble sleeping
- Irritability
- Panic attacks
- Depression
- Loss of eagerness and enthusiasm for life

Take a look at these symptoms, and realize that there are dozens of medications prescribed, artificial to the human body, dense with side-effects and nutrient depletions which could be eliminated or avoided with proper nutritional and hormonal balance.

Estrogen(s)

One of the biggest points of confusion and misconceptions in medicine is the fact that there is not just one estrogen. There are actually 3 main estrogens, each with different activities and affinity for different receptors. Estrogen works together with all the other hormones, although one big area we look at is estrogen's' relationship with progesterone.

To simplify it, estrogen makes tissue grow, and progesterone steps in and tells the tissue to grow healthy, as well as to die healthy. This is why estrogen cream is often used vaginally to increase vaginal wall thickness, it promotes the tissues growth and thickness.

The counter side to the growth is if it is done in an imbalanced fashion. For instance, if someone had too high of estrogen levels, especially in comparison to progesterone levels, what is known as estrogen dominant, than tissue growth could be hyper-stimulated, thus leading to fears that estrogen can influence tumor growth and be related to cancer.

Another very important point is that estrogen should not be taken orally, the optimum root of delivery is trans-dermally (through the skin) due to the nutrient depletions oral estrogen can cause including B vitamins, Vitamin C, CoQ10, Calcium, Vitamin E, Magnesium, Selenium, Zinc and others. Oral estrogen can lead to increase blood pressure, increase triglycerides, contribute to gallstones, can elevate liver enzymes, can decrease growth hormone, interrupt tryptophan and serotonin metabolism (possibly leading to prescribing of unnecessary antidepressants), increase carbohydrate cravings and weight gain.

Functions Of Estrogens

- Helps to prevent Alzheimer's disease
- Increases your metabolic rate
- Improves insulin sensitivity
- Regulates body temperature
- Helps prevent muscle damage
- Helps maintain muscle
- Helps regulate your sleep
- Reduces your risk of cataracts
- Helps maintain the elasticity of your arteries
- Dilates your small arteries
- Increase blood flow
- Inhibits platelet stickiness
- Decreases the accumulation of plaque on your arteries
- Enhances magnesium uptake and utilization
- Maintains the amount of collagen in your skin
- Decreases blood pressure
- Decreases LDL (bad cholesterol) and prevents its oxidation
- Helps maintain your memory
- Increases reasoning and new ideas
- Helps with fine motor skills
- Increases the water content of your skin and is responsible for its thickness and softness
- Enhances the production of nerve-growth factor
- Increases HDL (good Cholesterol)

- Reduces the overall risk of heart disease
- Decreases lipoprotein A (a risk factor for heart disease)
- Acts as a natural calcium channel blocker to keep your arteries open
- Enhances energy
- Improves your mood
- Increases concentration
- Maintains bone density
- Increases sexual interest
- Reduces homocysteine (a risk factor for heart disease)
- Decreases wrinkles
- Protects against macular degeneration
- Decreases your risk of colon cancer
- Helps prevent tooth loss
- Aids in the formation of neurotransmitters in your brain such as serotonin which decreases depression, irritability, anxiety, and pain sensitivity

Once again, look at this list of functions and benefits and ask yourself, how many unnecessary prescriptions are dispensed, only treating symptoms, artificial to the human body, dense with side-effects and nutrient depletions which could be eliminated or avoided with proper nutritional and hormonal balance.

The 3 Estrogens

There are three main estrogens; estrone (E1), estradiol (E2), and estriol (E3). The body looks to have a balance between the three of these, and each one has different attributes and benefits.

Estrone (E1)

Estrone is the main estrogen that the female body makes in menopause. For this reason, practitioners often do not find a necessity to add it to hormone replacement therapy regimens. High levels of estrone can stimulate breast and uterine tissue and many believe it can lead to an increased risk of breast and uterine cancer.

Estradiol (E2)

Estradiol is the strongest estrogen that your body produces. It is estimated to be 12 stronger than estrone and 80 times stronger than estriol. Before menopause it is the main estrogen that the body produces, and after menopause experiences the biggest decline leading to issues of bone, heart, and even brain health. High levels of estradiol are associated with an increased risk of breast and uterine cancer which is important to note since this is the common estrogen prescribed in conventional medicine.

Estriol (E3)

Estriol has a much weaker stimulating effect on the breast and the uterine lining than estrone or estradiol. Do you remember when I said that estrogens make tissue grow and that's why a physician will prescribe it topically to increase the thickness of the uterine lining? Well, often estriol is chosen as a compounded prescription because it gives the desired effects with less risk of over stimulation. Another very interesting fact is that estriol has been shown not to promote breast cancer and there exists mounting evidence that it protects against it, actually being used as treatment in some studies. Even though the less stimulating effects of estriol seem to offer many great benefits, estriol does not have the bone, heart, or brain protection of estradiol, and this is why a combination of estradiol and estriol is often prescribed.

Estrogen Metabolism

So far we have discussed estrogens as well as 3 main estrogens; estrone, estradiol, and estriol. It turns out that's not all there is to the estrogen story.

The estrogens are further metabolized (broken down) into 3 main estrogen metabolites that account for good and bad actions in the body. This means that if our body is creating too many 'bad' metabolites, than negative consequences can result. On the other hand, if we are proactive through actions of a proper diet, supplementation, and proper testing to ensure our bodies are influencing the good metabolite pathways, it is one of the most powerful measures of preventative health we can provide ourselves.

The three major metabolites of estrogen are:

1. 2-hydroxyestrone

2. 16-hydroxyestrone

3. 4-hydroxyestrone

2-hydroxyestrone is also known as the "good estrogen" metabolite. It does not stimulate cells, thus avoiding further damage to DNA and lead to tumor growth. It also comes with a 'protective' or 'blocking' action which means that it blocks stronger estrogens from locking on to estrogen receptors. Thus it prevents excessive stimulation, leading it to be considered anti-cancerous.

16-Hydroxyestrone is the metabolite known as the "bad estrogen" metabolite. This metabolite is much more active and powerful with a greater stimulatory effect than the 2 and the 4-hydroxyestrones (and where 4-hydroxyestrone is believed to have some carcinogenic activity, it is considered to be a minor pathway so we will focus on the 2 and 16-hydroxyestrones.)

Where the 2-hydroxyestrone prevents other stronger estrogens from binding to receptor sites, the 16-hydroxyestrone binds very strongly to receptors inside the cells that can be very stimulatory and increase the rate of DNA synthesis and cell multiplication. On top of all this, 16-hydroxyestrone actually permanently binds to the estrogen receptors where other hormones and metabolites bind only temporarily. Add to this the fact that

16-hydroxyestrone is much stronger and more stimulating and is associated with a higher rate of cancer.

Being that the 2-hydroxyestrones and the 16-hydroxyestrones are the 2 most powerful, one good, one bad; we can measure the ratio to get an assessment of carcinogenic risk. For those looking to test this ratio, there is a urine test known as estronex in which more information can be obtained at Metametrix laboratories.

From a preventative mode there are risk factors which we know can raise the 16-hydroxyestrone metabolite. Obesity increases the actions of estrogens thus the 16-hydroxyestrone and so due xenoestrogens. Xenoestrogens are chemicals that mimic estrogenic activity at the receptor sites to increase stimulation, as well as to influence the ratio of 2/16 hydroxyestrogen which may account for an increase of certain cancers like breast cancer. Sources of xenoestrogens are pesticides, hormones fed to animals, plastics and cosmetics.

There are various ways to help raise the 2-hydroxystrone levels (good metabolite) thus reducing the risk factors mentioned above, including: Moderate exercise, consuming cruciferous vegetables such as; broccoli, Brussels sprouts, cabbage, cauliflower, collard, bok choy, horseradish, kale, mustard seed, radishes, rutabaga, turnip, and watercress and flax. Supplements such as kudzu, indole-3-Cardinol and DIM (diindolymethane), a high protein diet, omega-3-fatty acids, and Vitamins B6, B12, and folate are all important to support the 2-Hydroxyestrone pathway.

Progesterone

Progesterone is a sex hormone that is made primarily from the ovaries before menopause, and after menopause some is made in the adrenal glands. As you will see, aging is a natural cause of progesterone deficiency, although there are other factors that could cause or influence lower progesterone levels such as stress, medications such as antidepressants, diets high in sugar and saturated fat, deficiencies of Vitamins A, B6, C, and zinc.

Hormonal therapy with progesterone takes place when we see that there is deficiency of progesterone, either later in life during peri-menopause and menopause, or even during the menses years with a condition known as luteal phase deficiency.

As we spoke about above on estrogen, there should be a healthy balance between estrogen and progesterone, but over time due to progesterone deficiency the balance becomes out of whack. This is something that is called estrogen dominance. Estrogen dominance can lead to issues such as fibroids and endometriosis. Estrogen tells tissue to grow, and progesterone's job is to tell the tissue to grow healthy and die healthy. This alone is a reason why estrogen should not be given unopposed by progesterone which is often done in conventional medicine.

Eventually after years of dealing with endometriosis or uterine fibroid's, a woman might end up in surgery for a hysterectomy. A full hysterectomy is where both the uterus and ovaries are removed.

Remember how I said in the beginning that progesterone is produced by the ovaries? By removing the ovaries in the case of a full hysterectomy, or oophorectomy, we are then putting the body at an even greater imbalance of estrogen to progesterone. In a full hysterectomy, the body's primary and major source of progesterone production is removed, but the body can still create estrogen via fat tissue, hair follicles and adrenal glands. This is not to say it's therapeutic estrogen for bones, heart and brain health, although it is mainly estrone which can be stimulating to tissue, thus the balance with progesterone is critical.

What often happens in conventional medicine in the case of a hysterectomy is that a woman is given more estrogen which really only calms the symptoms and adds fuel to the fire, while the imbalance still exists. What would be a better option is proper measurement, and balancing with progesterone and estrogen if needed.

It's important not to confuse bio-identical progesterone with the synthetic version, called progestin. Progestin is very different from natural progesterone. Where a progestin might have similar activity at the vaginal tissue, it works completely the opposite in other parts of the body. This is important to understand considering that we have progesteron[e] on practically all cells in our body.

Progestin's can be found in birth-control pills, conventional horm[one] replacement medications such as Provera®, Prempro®, and other prescription medications. The use of birth control for prevention of conception is a risk-benefit issue, although birth-control pills should not be considered therapy for hormonal balance.

Let me share with you some of the major difference between progestin's and progesterone. Side-effects of Progestin's (just a partial list): Increased appetite, weight gain, fluid retention, irritability, depression, decreased sexually interest, insomnia, acne, does not balance estrogen, breast tenderness, stops the protective effects estrogen has on the heart, increases LDL (bad cholesterol), and decreases HDL (good cholesterol).

To the contrary, some of the benefits of progesterone not seen in progestin's include: helps balance estrogen, supports sleep, has a natural calming effect, lowers high blood pressure, lowers cholesterol, may protect against breast cancer, helps your body utilize and eliminate fats, may protect against breast cancer, increases metabolic rate, helps building of bone, supports thyroid function, normalizes libido, increases the beneficial effects of estrogens on blood vessel dilation and atherosclerotic plaques, natural diuretic and natural anti-depressant.

There are many symptoms of decreased progesterone levels and since we mentioned that almost every cell in the body has progesterone receptors, you will see that the symptoms are far and wide including; anxiety, depression, irritability, mood swings, insomnia, pain and inflammation, osteoporosis, decreased HDL (good cholesterol) and excessive menstruation.

As I mentioned, it is optimal to have one's progesterone levels tested, although you can acquire bio-identical progesterone over the counter, without a prescription. Many people choose this option, and it is important to note that too much of a good thing can be a bad thing. Progesterone cream can build up in the tissues, like a sponge, and lead to too much progesterone in the body. If this is the case it can lead to increased fat storage, increases cortisol, increases insulin resistance, increases appetite, increases carbohydrate cravings, relaxes

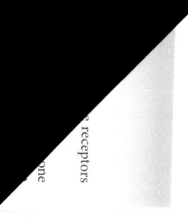

This can cause bloating, fullness, and constipa-
;allstones), suppresses immune system, causes
causes your ligaments to relax and can cause
hips, and can decrease natural levels of growth

Testosterone

Testosterone, "the guy hormone," is actually a very important hormone to follow in both men and women. Testosterone is considered an
androgen and shares the family with DHEA, and androstenedione.

Men actually have a change in life much akin to a woman's menopause,
which is aptly called andropause. This is the time where their androgen
levels have decreased, leading to symptoms and even affecting disease states
linked to sub-par levels of hormones such as testosterone.

Testosterone, in men is made primarily in the testicles and to a lesser
extent in the adrenal glands; for women, primarily in the ovaries, and a lesser amount in the adrenal glands as well.

The 'norm' for testosterone levels is actually quite broad, so falling in
to the 'norm' but still exhibiting levels of low androgen levels should be further investigated. In a perfect world we would have gotten a reading of our
testosterone levels somewhere around the age of 20 years old or so when
our levels are at their peak, to give us a marker to work off of that is more
individualistic as we age.

For instance, someone might naturally have been running at a level in
the high 700's during their late teens and twenties, but when they hit their
50's or so, levels could be precipitously lower, such as in the 300's. Where a
reading in the 300's might be in the 'normal' range, being void of over half
the amount of testosterone that one once had is not normal, and if symptomatic dysfunction exists...this should be further examined.

The customization and individualization continues from assessment to
treatment. Like other hormonal therapies, testosterone replacement is not a
one size fits all approach. That is why through proper symptom and testing

assessment a preparation can be customized specifically for you, to help you be the best you can be.

It is also important to understand that there are other reasons for low testosterone besides menopause and andropause including; childbirth, chemotherapy, surgery, adrenal stress or burnout, endometriosis, depression, psychological trauma, birth control pills, cholesterol lowering medications called HMG-CoA-redutase inhibitors, such as Lipitor®, Mevacor®, Zocor®, Pravachol®, and others .

So, what does testosterone do for us? Testosterone is responsible for increasing sexual interest (a major complaint during the times of menopause and andropause), increases emotional well-being, self-confidence, and motivation. Testosterone increases muscle mass and strength, it helps maintain memory, increases skin tone as well as decreases excess body fat. Testosterone helps with prevention of osteoporosis by decreasing bone deterioration and helps maintain bone strength. Testosterone also elevates norepinephrine in the brain, which is what medications do in the class of drugs known as tricyclic antidepressants such as Elavil® (amitriptyline) as well as another popular antidepressant known as Wellbutrin ® (buproprion).

When people are low on testosterone, common symptoms are muscle wasting, weight gain, decreased energy, low self-esteem, decreased HDL (good cholesterol), decreased sex drive, depression, poor skin elasticity, thinning dry hair, and anxiety.

There are various ways to increase testosterone levels, obviously by supplementing with bio-identical testosterone itself. If this is done it is recommended to measure testosterone levels regularly as well as to monitor symptoms. It might also be a good idea to measure estrogen levels, even in men, because with testosterone therapy a process called aromatization can occur, which will pool the testosterone into estrogen. This is often represented, especially in males by enlargement of breast tissue. People who are overweight have a higher chance of increasing this estrogen pathway, and there are natural supplements and medications known as aromatase inhibitors to help stop this from happening.

Other than using testosterone itself, there are other ways to support ones testosterone levels such as decreasing calorie intake, increasing protein in your diet, amino acids arginine, leucine, glutamine, and supplements such as tribulis, zinc, exercise, losing weight if overweight, and stress reduction techniques.

It is important to recognize that someone can suffer from increased testosterone, especially women. Aside from supplementing, reasons for increased testosterone usually revolve around over production of androgens such as DHEA and testosterone, often through adrenal glands (often related to stress), and a hormone imbalance related to health conditions such as PCOS which is often related to insulin resistance and metabolic syndrome.

Symptoms of elevated testosterone, regardless of the cause include; anxiety, depression, fatigue, hypoglycemia (low blood sugar), salt and sugar cravings, agitation, anger and mood swings, facial hair (in females), acne/oily skin, increase in insulin resistance, decrease in HDL (good cholesterol), irregular periods, fluid retention, hair loss or unwanted hair growth.

Testing For Hormones

In the last section we mentioned the best way to test for adrenal hormones such as cortisol and DHEA is through salivary testing. It turns out that saliva testing for other hormones is also the preferred method, allowing all hormones to be tested at the same time. Salivary testing will allow someone to test all three estrogens, estrone, estradiol, and estriol, as well as progesterone, and testosterone, in addition to the cortisol and DHEA. Combining all of these together will allow the practitioner to provide an assessment of the relationships between the hormones. For instance, rising cortisol levels can steal from progesterone since they are made up of similar material being steroidal hormones. One can see relationships between falling testosterone and rising estrogen which can lead to aromatization, one of the precursors and aggravators to estrogen induced problems.

And where this assessment gives a snap picture on what is happen now in one's life, what is even of more value is to have this test done on a regular basis, every 6 months to a year, to gain assessment on trends, how the hormones are behaving; rising or falling, especially while someone is on hormone replacement therapy.

A Word On Hot Flashes

The western style medicine way of dealing with hot flashes via prescription has been to dowse with estrogen via a pill or a patch. This has tapered off a bit in recent years due to the awareness of estrogen dominant cancers and other issues. This is often only a symptomatic treatment and when done out of balance might only add fuel to the fire.

Remember how I talked about estrogen dominance? Most people, due to the increasing rates of people being overweight and even obese, are already estrogen dominant since fat tissue is an estrogen factory.

Thus you might calm a hot flash, but you might also be adding some unwanted and unnecessary additional estrogen dominance.

If your doctor prescribes estrogen it should be done with proper management and most likely with the opposing prescribing with progesterone to help balance the effect.

Due to many of the estrogen side-effects which often come when proper balance is not provided, many doctors have begun prescribing certain anti-depressants to treat hot flashes. Once again, we are avoiding the root cause, avoiding proper balance, and bringing to the table the downfalls of antidepressant medication therapy which you will read more about in chapter 18, Brain Benders.

This leads us to a plethora of over the counter natural supplements. Some work and some don't. Most of them exert a week estrogenic activity, and when they don't work it's usually due to one or more other reasons.

When I talk to someone who describes their hot flashes coming on like a storm, I often think adrenals. When your adrenals are running inefficient or suppressed, hot flashes can be the result, and no matter how much attention you give to estrogen and progesterone, you might still be missing the boat. Thyroid is another hormonal system that when in balance can help with someone's hormonal fluctuations such as hot flashes.

Lastly, we cannot forget about detox, especially the liver and gallbladder area. Whether it's due to the body's natural hormones or hormones added via medication therapy, the liver and gallbladder work to detoxify the hormones and their metabolites. I have seen time and time again, that by addressing this area through liver and gallbladder cleanses, one can effectively alleviate their hot flashes. Regular detoxification can provide a measure of preventative wellness to help the body eliminate built up hormones and hormone metabolites which can cause further problems.

When a client asks for a point and shoot solution for hot flashes, this is what I often tell them:

- Genibalance from Pure Encapsulations
- If hot flashes come on like a storm, add Relora for adrenal support
- If still need support, encourage balanced hormonal work-up from a qualified practitioner.

Hormonal Checklist

1. Find a practitioner who is trained and experienced in proper bio-identical hormonal balance. Conventional medical and pharmaceutical schooling is based on synthetic hormone utilization, not natural to the human body. See the reference section on our website at www.wholepharmacy.com. Conventional education tends to isolate the hormonal systems, where for best assessment; they should be looked at in relation to one another.

2. To test is best. Proper testing of hormones will allow a practitioner to dial in ones needs most effectively and efficiently.

3. Bio-Identical Hormones. Whole Pharmacy recommends if hormonal restoration is to be done, to do so with hormones which are bio-identical to what the body produces. These can be found at compounding pharma-

cies, which we provide more information in the reference section of our website, www.wholepharmacy.com

4. To be hormonally sound, it helps to be nutritionally sound. It's a complete game, hormones are not miracles, although they are our body's great communicators and work more efficiently when we provide a nutritionally healthy and balanced base.

5. Avoid estrogen and testosterone orally when possible. Oral estrogen therapy depletes numerous nutrients from your body, and oral testosterone is poorly absorbed. Optimal and efficient utilization of estrogen and testosterone is through transdermal usage, such as creams, patches, and sometimes pellets can be of benefit. This allows for lower dosages to achieve optimal levels of hormones.

6. Do not take estrogen without the opposition of progesterone. As we spoke of earlier, estrogen and progesterone work in balance, progesterone helps the tissues that estrogen stimulates to grow healthy and to die healthy. Many conventional practitioners will prescribe estrogen only therapy in an attempt to only quiet symptoms, even without measuring levels; this is not proper hormonal balance.

7. Diet. Refer to the chapter 7 for the backbone of a healthy diet, and when speaking of hormonal balance it is important to limit the amount of refined foods, sugars, flours and caffeine laden foods.

8. Understand that as we are becoming hormonally exhausted at an earlier age, women can often use the help of natural progesterone. As mentioned above, progesterone takes a hit from chronic stress and the body's need to keep creating cortisol, as well as the estrogen dominant factors we have in our society, from increased fat mass to estrogen stimulating toxins in our foods and our environments.

See also: Adrenal, Thyroid, and Detoxification.

Chapter 13
Thyroid – The Most Misunderstood Gland in Medicine

Subclinical hypothyroidism is probably one of the most under diagnosed and mismanaged issues of health. This is a big deal given the fact that there are more symptoms associated with thyroid imbalance than practically any other disease or condition. The reasons for such underdiagnoses or assessment are simple. (1) Often practitioners will not look at the whole thyroid picture by not taking into account all thyroid markers which should be tested. (2) Often a practitioner will recognize that a patient might still have low thyroid symptoms, although if thyroid testing says they are normal they do not go the extra mile to get to the root of the problem. (3) Lastly, it is important to realize that all hormones work together in a symphony like fashion, and by not addressing imbalances of hormones and even medication therapy, people often fall through the cracks with thyroid disease.

The thyroid has many roles in the body. Thyroid activity regulates energy and heat production, helps promote tissue repair and development, stimulates protein synthesis, increase utilization of carbohydrates and fats, stimulates appetite and movement/digestion of foods, plays a critical role in the utilization of vitamins and nutrients, increases the number of mitochondria (energy powerhouses of our cells), has many roles related to blood flow, hormone excretion, oxygen utilization and sexual function.

Symptoms of and conditions related to low thyroid activity (hypothyroidism) include:

- Depression
- Weight gain
- Constipation
- Headaches
- Brittle nails
- Rough, dry skin
- Depression
- Menstrual irregularities
- PMS
- Fluid retention
- Poor circulation
- Elbow keratosis
- Diffuse hair loss
- Slow speech
- Anxiety/Panic attacks
- Decreased memory
- Inability to concentrate
- Muscle and joint pain

- Reduced heart rate
- Slow movements
- Morning stiffness
- Puffy face
- Swollen eyelids
- Decreased sexual interest
- Cold intolerance
- Cold hands and feet
- Swollen legs, feet, hands, abdomen
- Insomnia
- Fatigue
- Low body temperature
- Hoarse, husky voice
- Low blood pressure
- Muscle weakness
- Agitation
- Sparse, coarse, dry hair
- Dull facial expression
- Yellowish color of the skin
- Muscle cramps
- Drooping eyelids
- Carpel tunnel syndrome
- High cholesterol

Once again, look at this list of symptoms and conditions of low thyroid levels and ask yourself, how many unnecessary prescriptions are dispensed, only treating symptoms, artificial to the human body, dense with side-effects and nutrient depletions which could be eliminated or avoided with proper nutritional and hormonal balance.

Thyroid Hormones

Now what I would like to do is talk about the main thyroid hormones and address what issues can lead to suppressed thyroid production or activity. The body produces two primary thyroid hormones, T3 (liothyronine) and T4 (levothyroxine). T4 is 80% of the Thyroid glands production. Most T4 is converted to T3 in the liver and kidneys. T3 is 4 to 5 times more active than T4.

T4 is created in the body by 2 primary ingredients, iodine and the amino acid tyrosine. In addition to deficiencies in tyrosine and iodine, other nutritional deficiencies which can lead to decreased T4 (levothyroxine) production include: Zinc, Copper, Vitamins A, B2, B3, B6, and C.

As I mentioned above, T4 is converted to T3 in a healthy, efficient working body, although there are many reasons why T4 might not convert to T3 as it should.

- Nutritional factors that can suppress the ability to convert T4 to T3 (thus low thyroid activity) include; deficiencies in iodine, iron, selenium, zinc, vitamins A, B2, B6, B12, inadequate protein intake, high carbohydrate diets, and starvation.

- There are many other health conditions which can lead to decreased conversion of T4 to T3 such as stress, elevated cortisol levels, even suppressed cortisol and DHEA production, chronic illness, diabetes, decreased kidney or liver function this too can inhibit the conversion of T4 to T3.

- Prescription medications can lead to a suppressed conversion of T4 to T3 including; beta blockers, birth control pill, estrogen, lithium, phenytoin, theophylline, and chemotherapy.

- One area that must be looked at if someone's thyroid tests are normal although they still have many hypothyroid symptoms is toxins. Toxins can impact the thyroid in a way that they can prevent thyroid hormone from stimulating the thyroid gland as they should and there are numerous toxins we must be aware of including; fluoride, lead, mercury, cadmium, pesticides, radiation, dioxins, PCB's, phthalate's (chemicals in plastics.)

It is important to mention that adrenal support might often be needed, especially when starting prescription thyroid therapy. We speak about a holistic view and this includes recognizing that hormones work optimally in a balanced supportive environment. I have seen many times someone's symptoms of adrenal suppression, which is similar to low thyroid symptoms, get worse with the addition of thyroid medication. The up regulating of the metabolism could be too much for the weakened adrenals to handle, much like constantly revving an old engine on high RPM's.

About Iodine

Iodine is basically food for the thyroid and is responsible for approximately 60% of thyroid hormone production. As a natural supplement, iodine has gained increased interest over the last decade or so based off the numerous benefits it has for not just thyroid, but prostate, breast tissues, immunity and more. Where the current RDA of 150 mcg has found to be sufficient for the thyroid, at least to keep goiters at bay, studies suggest larger amounts are needed for different tissues of the body. It is also important to understand that not all forms of iodine are the same and different types of iodine will concentrate in different tissues and glands within the body.

If you look at a multivitamin or iodine supplement for the thyroid you will often see that it has potassium iodide, potassium iodide has a strong affinity to the thyroid gland.

Aside from potassium iodide being used for thyroid health, iodine preparations have many other uses supportive to one's health due to iodine's antibacterial, anticancer, antiparasitic, and antiviral properties. Iodine is a toxin fighter, protecting the thyroid gland from dangerous toxins such as fluoride, bromide and radioactive iodine. Iodine is needed for proper immune system function, production of all hormones, and has been used to treat fibrocystic breasts and ovarian cysts. Iodine deficiency can lead to goiters, thyroid nodules, mental retardation, infertility, and child and infant mortality. The iodine which is used in supplementation is either in the form of straight iodine, potassium iodide, or combinations of both.

Historically, receiving the benefits of iodine through supplementation was problematic due to the fact that iodine itself is not very soluble in water. This made it difficult to get iodine into a solution which was water based. Then in 1829, Dr. Jean Lugol discovered that potassium iodide added to water increased the solubility of iodine. This led to Dr. Lugol to create and begin using a solution for infections known as Lugols solution, which was a mixture of 5% iodine and 10% potassium iodide in water.

The combination of iodine and its reduced form, iodide, led to another benefit and is a major reason why certain iodine preparations utilize such combinations today. Different tissues of the body actually prefer one, or both of these forms of iodine.

Earlier I mentioned the thyroid has affinity for potassium iodide, iodine itself is concentrated much more efficiently in areas such as prostate gland and breast tissue. Thus using a product that is purely potassium iodide might not give you the benefits you are looking for in the prostate and breast regions of the body. For reasons of supporting your overall health and taken on a daily regimen, combination products that utilize both iodine and potassium iodide is what is recommended.

Foods With High Iodine Content

Much of the growing interest in higher than RDA iodine doses have come about after realizing that cultures who have diets which are high in iodine rich foods have lower rates of breast cancer, prostate cancer, heart disease, thyroid disease and others. For example, the average Japanese diet consists on average of approximately 1 mg daily of iodine, which is 10 times greater than the average American diet.

It is important to note, that this 1 mg number is contested depending on one's school of thought. Many will say the average daily dose of the

Asian cultures is up to 12.5 mg's daily of iodine, thus has spurred over the counter supplements in the ranges of 12.5 mg's per dosage. Where these high dose supplements can adequately be used to treat someone's thyroid and other health issues, I only recommend a dose this high to be taken when adequately tested for iodine levels and under the guidance of a practitioner. Otherwise I recommend a combination iodine/potassium iodide or whole food iodine supplement with sources such as kelp, bladder wrack and dulce in levels of around 1 mg daily, as well as incorporating these foods into your diet. It is also important to note that too much iodine can lead to hyperthyroidism and even hypothyroidism.

Hypo-Thyroid Targeted Nutrients

Aside from iodine and tyrosine, there are numerous other supplements which have been shown to help with thyroid efficiency; below are some of my favorites with descriptions of the benefits they may provide.

Coleus- Enhances the efficiency at binding sites for thyroid hormone to the thyroid gland.

Cordyceps- In addition to supporting the adrenal glands, increases oxygen utilization which many hypothyroid patients deal with due to suppressed metabolic activity.

Ashwagandha- Supports the conversion of T4 to T3 and provides adaptogenic adrenal support.

Guggul- Stimulates the thyroid gland which might increase production, thus this is not to be used in patients on thyroid hormone therapy or those who are hyper-thyroid, unless being properly tested and monitored.

Thyroid Glandulars- Recommend to be sourced only from brucellosis free areas' such as in New Zealand and may not be recommended in cases of high thyroid antibodies.

Testing

I mentioned previously that one of the reasons people often fall through the cracks is that they are not adequately tested, thus not assessed completely for thyroid health. What happens in many areas of the country is that a doctor will only test for T4 and TSH. TSH is known as thyroid stimulating hormone, and even in medical literature is recommended only to be used as a screening tool and not a diagnostic tool. This means that if TSH is normal and someone still has low thyroid symptoms, the practitioner should dig further, opposed to assessing the thyroid activity as normal when it still might not be.

T4 is needed to convert to T3 for optimal thyroid activity, although often it is not. When a practitioner only tests T4 and not T3, a T4 might be normal and a T3 low, and it would go unnoticed, thus especially in the event where low thyroid symptoms are present, testing T3 as well as some other factors is critical. This is why we recommend for optimal thyroid assessment, a complete thyroid panel as described below.

Conversely, someone might actually have low T4 and high T3 levels. Thus, if someone is only tested for T4, then adding thyroid medication might then lead to even higher levels of T3, giving the patient symptoms of hyperthyroidism.

Complete Thyroid Panel

1. TSH (thyroid stimulating hormone) - Is made in you pituitary gland located in your brain. Your body releases this when it feels more thyroid hormone is needed by the body.

2. T4 (thyroxine) - Is made in your thyroid gland and accounts for more than 80% of the thyroid glands production. T4 is then changed into the more active T3 in the liver or kidneys.

3. T3 (triiodothyronine)-Is 5 times more active than T4, although can be low due to a decreased conversion ability from T4.

4. **Reverse T3-** Can be converted from T4, when in excessive amounts often due to prolonged stress. This is a biologically inactive form of T3 and has no effect on metabolism.

5. **Thyroid Anti-bodies-** If your antibodies are too high it can prevent the thyroid hormone from attaching to the thyroid receptors...no matter how high the levels. These levels can be elevated due to infection, inflammation or trauma to one's system.

Thyroid Checklist

1. Get adequate testing such as a Complete Thyroid Panel, as well as iodine testing as mentioned above.

2. Thyroid begins and ends with iodine. Whether you are on thyroid replacement medication or not, iodine can be of benefit. If working with an experienced practitioner one might go on high dose iodine, in products such as Iodoral. If not going the route of high dose iodine, taking an equivalent amount of iodine consumed by cultures with rich iodine content in their foods of around 1 mg daily can be beneficial. I like to recommend Vinco's Liposomal Liquid Iodine which provides a combination potassium iodide and natural iodine from kelp and dulce seaweed. Liposomal Liquid Iodine comes in a great tasting liquid which allows customized dosing. I recommend people to start out with .25 ml or less to provide around 1 to 3 mg of daily iodine. Keep in mind, when working with an experienced practitioner, dosages can go higher.

3. Thyroid support supplements can add a tremendous benefit. They provide the nutrients, cofactors and herbs to support a healthy thyroid production and metabolism. Two of my favorites are Thyroid Synergy from Designs for Health and Thyroid Support Complex from Pure Encapsulations.

See also: Adrenal, Hormones (especially progesterone if female), Nutritional Deficiency, and Detoxification health and support.

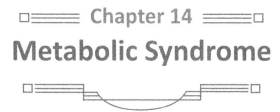

Chapter 14
Metabolic Syndrome

The Perfect Storm of Heart Disease and Diabetes

Metabolic Syndrome is a grouping of disease states and conditions which are highly preventable and could literally sink our healthcare system if we do not right our course. What I would like you to walk away from this with is that in almost all cases it is very preventable, medications do not come without risk, and there are what could be complements or even better options through natural medicine.

Metabolic Syndrome is a culmination of risk factors and disease states including abdominal obesity, insulin resistance, type II diabetes, hypertension, and dyslipidemia (cholesterol and triglycerides). Beyond cardiovascular disease and type 2 diabetes, metabolic syndrome has been implicated in driving almost every chronic disease and individuals with metabolic syndrome seemingly are susceptible to other conditions including; heart attacks, stroke, depression, arthritis, dementia, Alzheimer's disease, polycystic ovary syndrome (PCOS), infertility, fatty liver, cholesterol gallstones, asthma, sleep disturbances, obesity and some forms of cancer.

Insulin resistance is an epidemic in our society, it is often called pre-diabetes and the next step is type II diabetes. Insulin resistance is the result of one's body not effectively managing insulin and blood sugar. As sugar drops into the blood stream, one of insulin's' jobs is to escort it to a cell for energy, or to be stored for later use.

Too much sugar in the blood leads to too much insulin release, leading to insulin release overload. The end result, the body's is continually releasing too much insulin, and insulin being a fat storing hormone, leads to weight gain and other issues. Eventually the body runs out of its own insulin and then we have to go to insulin therapy.

Take a look around during the last 20 years at how obesity, insulin resistance and type II diabetes has exploded…it is no coincidence that Alzheimer's is not too far behind, and given the relationship many experts are calling this the next medical tsunami. *Alzheimer's disease is now being linked to metabolic syndrome and insulin resistance in what is being called Type 3 Diabetes,* also referred to as Brain Diabetes.

Type I, insulin dependent diabetes, is the result of an autoimmune condition where the body targets its own pancreas and cells that create insulin. This is about 5 to 10% of cases. Type II diabetes is practically totally preventable through diet and lifestyle although this accounts for 90 to 95% of diabetes cases. If society would just drop the pop and the carbohydrate laden, processed foods and make the switch back to real healthy foods it would be amazing what would happen.

The numbers of the escalating metabolic syndrome, related conditions morbidity, and financials are startling:

- Type 1 diabetes rose 23% among young people during the first nine years of the 21st century, while type 2 increased by 21%.

- About $174 billion was spent to treat diabetes in the U.S. last year, while chronic diseases in total accounted for about 75% of total healthcare spending (majority related to metabolic syndrome).

- Some models forecast the number of people with diabetes doubling to between 50 million and 55 million by 2025 from 26 million in the U.S. today, he said.

- One in two Americans are now pre-diabetic or diabetic.

- 2/3 adults over weight, greater than 1/3 obese

- In 1990, there was not a single state in the country where obesity was over 20%.

- Now in 2013, there is not a single state in the country where the obesity rate is under 20%.

- It is estimated that in 20 years ½ Americans will be clinically obese.

- Heart disease is the number one killer of adults in the United States.

- One in two people will die of heart disease

- The United States ranks last among 16 other developed countries in major health conditions including heart disease, diabetes and others, while at the same time spending the most money on health care.

Testing and Assessment

Given the risk factors for Metabolic Syndrome it is quite easy to assess, test and track your health and this allows you to take a proactive approach with lifestyle adjustments such as diet and possibly nutritional supplementation support.

Basic goals of any therapy for heart disease, metabolic syndrome and diabetes:

- Healthy Lipid levels
- Healthy Triglycerides
- Healthy Sugar and Insulin
- Provide antioxidants to prevent oxidation of lipids
- Reduce arteriosclerosis
- Reduce Inflammation

Below you will find a summary of some of the basic tests which can be done to help identify risk factors related to metabolic syndrome, heart disease and diabetes. After each test/risk factor you will see a list of natural supplements which can help reduce risk factors. You will notice that there are some usual suspects; this is what I love about nutritional therapies, supplements can often provide multiple benefits as you will see in regards to metabolic syndrome, cardiovascular health and diabetes.

Risk Factors and Tests

A quick word about cholesterol- Cholesterol has been vilified by the medical establishment, although one must understand the battle cry should not be "less is more," it should be about balance and the bigger picture. Below are just a few of the purposes which cholesterol serves:

- A pro-hormone, precursor to vitamin D3, the sex hormones, estrogen, progesterone, and testosterone, and the steroid hormones such as cortisol.
- Cholesterol is essential to the cell membranes of all of our cells, where it protects the cell not only from leaks like a bandage, but also from oxidation damage.
- While the brain contains only 2% of the body's weight, it houses 25% of the body's cholesterol. Cholesterol is vital to the brain for nerve signal transport.

- Cholesterol sulfate plays an important role in the metabolism of fats via bile acids, as well as in immune defenses against invasion by pathogenic organisms.

Additionally, many would argue that we are completely missing the boat on heart disease assessment by focusing primarily on cholesterol, what many call the cholesterol myth, recognizing that cholesterol is not the best prevention for heart disease.

The culprit of heart disease continually proves to be inflammation and the cascade of problems inflammation can cause. This is why below I focus additionally on other biomarkers such as C-reactive protein, Fibrinogen, Homocysteine, Lipoprotein A, Triglycerides, and others.

- **Total Cholesterol, LDL Cholesterol, HDL Cholesterol, and VLDL Cholesterol** – A standard cholesterol profile usually consists of measuring Total Cholesterol, LDL (Low Density Lipoprotein aka bad cholesterol,) and HDL (High Density Lipoprotein aka good cholesterol.) Where high levels of total cholesterol and LDL, and low levels of HDL have been associated with risk of cardiovascular disease- it's about balance. VLDL (Very-low-density lipoprotein) is a type of lipoprotein which contains the highest amount of triglyceride. Having a high VLDL level means you may have an increased risk of coronary artery disease, which can lead to a heart attack, high blood pressure or stroke.

What HDL and LDL Do:

HDL and LDL should be looked at as transporters; they carry cholesterol throughout the body. HDL carries cholesterol from the blood to the liver for elimination from the body; LDL carries cholesterol, nutrient dense fats, vitamin D and fat-soluble anti-oxidants to all the tissues of the body. By interfering with the production of LDL too much, you can reduce the bioavailability of all these nutrients to your body's cells.

(Supplements to help balance cholesterol: Berberine, Red Yeast Rice, Policosanol, Niacin, tocotrienols, Plant Sterols CoQ10, Chromium, fiber, Garlic, Magnesium, Fish Oil)

- **Triglycerides** -Triglycerides are the form that fat takes when it is being stored for energy in your body. Triglycerides, liked cholesterol, are vital for human life but unhealthy if at too high a level. Causes of high triglyceride levels can be soft drinks, fruit juice, a high fat diet, white bread, flour and sugar, birth control pills, alcohol, caffeine, and others.

(Supplements to help balance triglycerides- Chromium, CoEnzyme Q10, Fish Oil, Magnesium, Berberine, Carnitine, Niacin, Policosanol, Vitamin E)

- **Lipoprotein (A)** is a small cholesterol particle that can cause inflammation and clog blood vessels when present in the body in elevated levels. High Lipoprotein A levels can greatly increase a person's risk of developing heart disease. An interesting point is that taking statin drugs to lower your cholesterol can actually lead to an increase of Lipoprotein A in the body, thus almost by definition, anyone on a statin medication should have their Lipoprotein A levels tested.

(Supplements to help balance Lipoprotein A- CoQ10, Fish Oil, L-Carnitine, L-Lysine, L-Proline, Vitamin E, Vitamin C)

- **Homocysteine**- Homocysteine is an amino acid that promotes free radical production, as well as elevates triglyceride and cholesterol levels. Since homocysteine can lead to elevation of triglyceride and cholesterol levels, homocysteine should be tested in an individual with elevated cholesterol and triglycerides. Studies indicate that high homocysteine levels are directly related to strokes, peripheral vascular disease, and cardiovascular disease.

(Supplements to help balance Homocysteine- B6, B12, Folic Acid and Trimethlyglycine)

- **C - Reactive Protein** is a protein that is found in the blood. Its levels become elevated when the body detects an infection or need for inflammation. Elevated levels may also indicate future problems including cardiovascular disease and atherosclerosis due to persistent issues of inflammation.

(Supplements to help balance C-Reactive Protein- CoEnzyme Q10, Aged Garlic, Curcumin, Fish Oil, Green Tea, Vitamin E)

- **Fibrinogen-** Fibrinogen is a clot-promoting substance in your blood. Elevated levels of this molecule can cause a heart attack all by itself.

(Supplements to help balance Fibrinogen- Fish Oil, Aged Garlic, Vitamin E, Bromelain)

- **Blood Pressure** - If left untreated, hypertension can lead to cardiovascular disease as well as a wide variety of other life-threatening conditions, such as kidney damage and congestive heart failure. Several studies have proven that insulin resistance can cause increases in blood pressure and since elevated levels of insulin can cause atherosclerosis which directly affects the diameter of the inside of the blood vessels which can lead to high blood pressure, anyone with insulin resistance and high blood pressure should not ignore getting their insulin resistance in line.

  (Supplements to help balance blood pressure- Alpha Lipoic Acid, B Complex Vitamins, CoEnzyme Q10, Fish Oil, Aged Garlic, Magnesium, Vitamin D, Arginine, Calcium, Carnitine, Vitamin E, Zinc)

- **Hemoglobin A1c (HbA1c) and Fasting Blood Sugar** – Testing HbA1c provides the average blood sugar level over the past three months, including both fasting and post prandial levels. Due to the fact that blood sugar levels can vary considerably from day to day, HbA1c levels are considered to be a more reliable assessment to track one's blood sugar status. A consistent elevation of HbA1c levels can be indicative of loss of blood sugar control, a risk factor of diabetes.

Blood sugar levels do have their value. What equates to pre-diabetes has changed over the years. Researchers found that pre-diabetes based on the 1997 American Diabetes Association (ADA) definition of 110 to 125 mg/dl carried a 21% higher chance of stroke. Now many groups say that pre-diabetes should start at 100 mg/dl.

This suggests that there may be a 'threshold effect' with regard to the relationship between impaired fasting glucose and future stroke risk to the extent that the risk of a stroke only begins to rise at or above a fasting glucose level of 110 mg/dL. Thus one should not look at pre-diabetes as all the same, and should work to get numbers in line below 100 mg/dl.

(Supplements to help balance blood sugar- Alpha lipoic acid, B complex, CoEnzyme Q10, Fish Oil, Vitamin D, chromium, Fiber, Magnesium, berberine, biotin, bitter melon, Vanadium, Vitamin E)

- Fasting Insulin – Fasting insulin levels are a reliable way of measuring the degree of insulin resistance. Insulin resistance can further influence high blood sugar levels and other metabolic disturbances such as altered blood lipid profiles and high blood pressure.

(Supplements to help balance insulin- Alpha Lipoic Acid, B complex, Chromium, CoEnzyme Q10, Fish Oil, Fiber, Magnesium, Vitamin D, CLA, Vitamin E, Berberine)

- Thyroid- decreased T3 will lead to elevated levels of LDL (bad cholesterol). This is why it is important for your physician to provide a full thyroid panel (free T3, free T4, TSH, and Thyroid Anti-bodies), not just the T4 and TSH which is often the case.

- In addition there are innovative advancements in technology and assessment such as oxidative stress as well as arterial and endothelial health. The Cleveland Heart Lab and Pure Encapsulations Nutritional Company have come together to offer the Pure Heart Protocol, which addresses assessment of such risk factors and treatments through nutraceutical therapy. (www.pureheartprotocol.com)

I think our medical society is still caught up in the "let's deal with it when it happens," which is often too late. Disease states of metabolic syndrome are highly preventable if we take action at the right time, thus so many people do not have to reside themselves to handfuls of medications, lost days of work and school, and loss of health and freedom.

Additionally, it seems the conversation based on diabetes and conditions of metabolic syndrome are all about "what new drugs can we develop to treat the disease" after it happens. Shouldn't the conversation be about "let's focus on preventing these disease states or reversing the trend naturally before it's too late, and if we need to get some risk factors in line, let's do it in the safest and most beneficial way possible?"- This is not what's happening.

Take heart disease as an example. We already know that heart disease is the number one killer of both men and women, although a recent report found that the United States of America is unhealthier than 16 other developed countries. The report, which was compiled by the National Research Council and the Institutes of Medicine, found that, despite the fact that Americans spend the most money per year on healthcare, we're not healthier or living longer than other countries.

Of the health areas studied, Americans ranked worse than other countries in nine categories, including, among others, heart disease, obesity and diabetes. So heart disease is the number one killer, the U.S. is last in line of developed countries for heart health, the biggest focus on attacking heart disease in our medical system is cholesterol management, while the U.S. tests more cholesterol and dispenses more prescriptions for cholesterol lowering medications- And only ½ of people who die of heart attacks have high cholesterol. This is just one example in our western prescription based system of medicine where we are spending way too much money and people are staying sick and dying.

Common Prescription Drug Therapies for Metabolic Disorders

Given the number of disease state risk factors related to metabolic syndrome, there are numerous prescription drugs prescribed. It is important to realize that the goal of prescription therapy is help reduces someone's risk factors; it is often not without side-effects or other challenges. Below are some of the common drug therapies, as well as issues which have in the past or might present themselves. Here we will be focusing on the two main common risk factors of the metabolic syndrome umbrella based on drug classed prescribed; insulin/blood sugar medications and cholesterol lowering medications.

Diabetes Medications

Metformin

Metformin (Glucophage ®) is often the first drug of first choice for many conditions of diabetes, whether you are insulin resistant, pre-diabetic or have diagnosed diabetes. By many counts metformin is considered a "good drug" with a low side-effect profile, although it has been recognized that upwards of 30% of patients can experience B12 deficiency, often resulting in peripheral neuropathies. Additionally it can provide a stress on the kidneys, often a challenge in diabetics anyway, thus kidney function should be regularly monitored.

Researchers presenting at the American Diabetes Association Scientific Sessions summer 2012 noted that:

Chronic metformin use has been previously shown to be associated with vitamin B_{12} deficiency. Peripheral neuropathy is typically diagnosed as diabetic neuropathy, but this can also be a symptom of vitamin B_{12} deficiency.

Thiazolidinediones (Avandia and Actos)

Both Avandia® (rosiglitazone) and Actos® (pioglitazone) are in the family of diabetes medications known as thiazolidinediones. They work by increasing an individual's sensitivity to insulin, thus directly combating the insulin resistance. As we have seen in recent years, they do not come without their own downfalls or side-effects.

Avandia

Rosiglitazone (Avandia®) has been severely restricted in its prescribing due to a list of cardiac risk events it has shown to be responsible for. One study estimated that from 1999 to 2009, more than 47,000 people taking Avandia needlessly suffered a heart attack, stroke or heart failure, or died.

This has led the FDA to restrict the prescribing of rosiglitazone United States where patients will be allowed access to the medicine only if they and their doctors attest that they have tried every other diabetes medicine and that patients have been made aware of the drug's substantial risks to the heart. The guidelines continue to warn that because of the risk of serious side effects, rosiglitazone should only be used to treat people who are already taking the medication, or people whose blood sugar cannot be controlled with other medications and who have decided not to take pioglitazone for medical reasons.

In addition to the cardiac events, other side-effects include liver problems, and an increased possibility of breaking of bones, which are all enhanced risk factors and disease states for the diabetic population.

Actos

Pioglitazone (Actos®) also carries with it a black box warning for congestive heart failure and myocardial infarction and shares other side-effects with rosiglitazone including weight gain, liver problems, increased chance of breaking bones, and something unique to pioglitazone, an increase risk of developing bladder cancer.

DPP 4 Inhibitors

DPP 4 Inhibitors are a class of medications including Januvia (Sitagliptin), Onglyza (Saxagliptin), and Trajenta (Linagliptin) while a number of additional DPP-4 inhibitors are currently under development. These drugs are used either alone or in combination with other oral anti-hyperglycemic agents (such as metformin or a thiazolidinedione) for treatment of type II diabetes. As you will see, the side-effect profile to this drug is growing, such as a potential link to cancer.

Below are some studies brought to light by Dr. Joseph Mercola (www. mercola.com) which has indicated a connection of pancreatic, thyroid, colon, melanoma, and prostate cancer with DPP-4 inhibitors. Such studies include:

- A 2006 study found that "the use of DPPIV inhibitors together with GLP-2 led to increased proliferation as well as elevated migratory activity. Therefore, the use of DPPIV inhibitors could increase the risk of promoting an already existing intestinal tumor and may support the potential of colon cancer cells to metastasize"

- One 2008 study found that DPP-4 inhibitors may proteolytically inactivate local mediators involved in gliomagenesis (the formation and development of brain tumors). Another study published that same year linked the drug to prostate cancer

- In 2010, researchers concluded that "although the data on the effects of DPP-IV inhibitors in humans are scarce, the increased risk of infections and the tendency towards a higher incidence of some tumors fall in line with experimental evidence suggesting the possibility of their adverse immunological and oncological effects"

- According to a 2011 study in the journal *Gastroenterology* "data are consistent with case reports and animal studies indicating an increased risk for pancreatitis with glucagon-like peptide-1 based therapy. The findings also raise caution about the potential long-term actions of these drugs to promote pancreatic cancer, and DPP-4 inhibition to increase risk for all cancers"

- Earlier this year, researchers warned DPP-4 "is implicated in regulation of malignant transformation, promotion and further progression of cancer, exerting tumor-suppressing or even completely opposite - tumor-promoting activities.

Seeing how thes DPP-4's act in the body, tumor growth and expression should be no surprise. Keep in mind, that at any given time, anyone of us can have an active cancer, or a seed of cancer growing in our system. We rely on a very intelligent immune system to identify, address and suppress such activity before it gets out of control.

The way these drugs lower blood sugar is by inhibiting DPP-4. DPP-4 is an enzyme that, among other things, destroys a hormone, GLP-1. GLP-1 helps control blood sugar levels, thus when you inhibit DPP-4, GLP-1 levels to rise and blood sugars drop.

But here's the kicker, **DPP-4 is also a tumor suppressor,** *and when you inhibit it, cells that have become cancerous are no longer under the watchful eye of our immune system and essentially we lose one of our innate functions to inhibit tumor growth.*

Another issue I think most practitioners avoid looking at is that most of these drugs can have a negative influence on kidney health. Plus, drug's such as Januvia are often not effective enough, thus it is often recommended to be combined with other agents like metformin (further increase stress on kidneys) or a thiazolidinedione (thus opening up further cardiovascular risk factors, potential for weight gain, and osteoporosis- all of which are enhanced risk factors in the diabetic population without such medication therapy.)

Cholesterol Lowering Medications

HMG CoA Reductase Inhibitors - Statins

Since statins are the #1 class of drugs for lowering your cholesterol, we will focus primarily on this class of medications. As I mentioned earlier, the main focus on lowering cholesterol to prevent heart disease is outdated science, yet cholesterol lowering drugs are the number one weapon doctors will use and pharmacists will dispense in hopes to lower someone's chances of heart disease.

The studies are clear, statin drugs do nothing to prevent a heart attack in people who have no prior issue of heart disease. There is research showing that people who have had previous issues of heart disease can benefit from statin therapy, although the research is still not based on cholesterol. Take the Jupiter study for instance where it was concluded that a statin drug can prevent heart disease by its influence on a biomarker such as C Reactive Protein. This makes sense because as we said earlier, inflammation is a marker of heart disease which C Reactive Protein can identify. The argument exists though that inflammation can be reduced with diet and supplements while avoiding the side-effects and risks that come with statin drugs.

One of the risks is the depletion of CoQ10 which statin drugs can cause, which is a key nutrient for the mitochondria to create energy, as well as a powerful antioxidant. CoQ10 is critical for muscle health, and your heart is a muscle, thus depleting CoQ10 in the effort to lower cholesterol could be adding insult to injury. This is why it is often recommended while taking statins to supplement with a high quality Coenzyme Q10 supplement, although even with supplementation one must realize the challenges we are still creating for healthy aging of the mitochondria. To add insult to injury, statin drugs are not the only medications which deplete CoQ10. There are numerous drugs, and many used to treat disease states of metabolic syndrome such as blood pressure lowering medications, diuretics, diabetes medications and others, thus creating a snowball the affect.

Cognitive disorders are another problem and even the FDA has advised consumers and health care professionals of cognitive (brain-related) impairment, such as memory loss, forgetfulness and confusion, increased risk of diabetes (already a risk factor in this population), as well as muscle damage in patients who have taken statin drugs.

Integrative Steps for Radical Change

Yes, it is time to take health back into your own hands. Here are some simple tips to get or keep the ball rolling, regardless of your current state of health in regards to metabolic syndrome:

Diet- What to Eat

- Eat it if it grows on a plant eat it, if it's created in a plant, don't eat it.
- Whole Foods rich in phytonutrients.
- 8 to 10 servings of colorful vegetables every day- different colors, different beneficial attributes, phytonutrients, and antioxidants such as polyphenols.
- Healthy liquid choices- Green tea, pomegranate.
- Healthy proteins and lean animal protein- fish, turkey, chicken, buffalo, lean lamb, vegetables, nuts, beans, tofu.
- Good oils- olive, sesame, nut oils.
- Good fats- Omega 3 fatty acids, cold water wild salmon, sardines, herring, seaweed, coconut oil, nut butters.
- High fiber- whole beans, whole grains, nuts, seeds, vegetables.

- Low in saturated fats- grass fed beef (less sat fat).
- Good Carbohydrates- Low Glycemic, High Fiber.

Diet- What NOT to Eat

- Reduce or eliminate liquid calories, alcohol increases triglycerides (especially beer)
- Avoid white flour and white sugar
- Junk food, Soda pop, sugar or diet
- No hydrogenated fats, no trans fats, no margarine, shortening, processed oils
- Processed and refined foods and genetically modified foods (GMO)

Other Healthy Tips

- Keep blood sugar balanced- avoid spikes and valleys-protein with every meal, have breakfast every day (protein based).
- Never eat a carbohydrate alone- combine protein fats and proteins.
- Graze when you eat, don't allow yourself to get hungry- snacks every 3 to 4 hours.
- Don't eat before bed.
- Promoting regular physical activities appropriate for the individual's state of health. We are meant to move, not to be static.

After life-style and diet, nutritional supplementation can play a terrific role in modifying risk factors. If used in combination with medications, it is recommended to check with a knowledgeable physician or pharmacist as certain supplements can affect the metabolism and blood levels of medications, thus altering their activity.

Blood Pressure

Issues of elevated blood pressure might fall into the realm of metabolic syndrome, and sometimes not. There are actually a number of reasons for elevated blood pressure, and I believe oftentimes it might be numerous of reasons, not just one. Because of this, I will lightly address blood pressure, although will make related recommendations more in depth throughout this book.

Possible reasons for high blood pressure:

- Stress

- Dietary habits

- Heavy metal toxicities

- Nutritional depletions, often caused by medications to lower blood pressure. Magnesium deficiencies are a major culprit here due to depletions through food sources and medications.

- GMO foods- decrease the product of eNOS, thus limits the production of nitrous oxide, a natural vasodilator

Below you will find natural supplements which have shown benefits in multiple areas of metabolic syndrome. It is important to note that we recommend only the highest in quality of supplements.

Foundational Metabolic Support

- **Comprehensive Multi Vitamin-** A multivitamin will provide foundational support of vitamins, minerals and antioxidants. These are designed to provide the necessary cofactors nutritional support for a healthy metabolism. Some multivitamins will encompass adequate amounts of the other foundational support I mention below.

- **Omega 3 Essential Fatty Acids-** Essential fatty acids support the integrity of cell membrane to allow binding of insulin to receptors as well as nutrients such as glucose (blood sugar) to flow in and out. Omega 3 Fatty acids have shown to support healthy HDL and triglycerides, help lower blood pressure, decrease homocysteine, and support healthy platelet function.

- B Vitamins- B Complex vitamins help proper metabolism of protein, fats and carbohydrates, they can help metabolize glucose to provide a balance to blood sugar and insulin support, and provide a wide array of benefits depending on which B vitamin for many metabolic conditions.

- Magnesium- Magnesium increases the pancreas' response in hyperglycemia (high blood sugar) and supports insulin's' actions to reduce insulin resistance. Magnesium is a nutrient that 75% of North Americans are deficient in that can decrease total cholesterol, decrease triglycerides and LDL, and increase HDL.

- Fiber- Fiber has shown to decrease total cholesterol and LDL, and can help slow the glycemic (sugar) response and insulin stimulation. The problem is most diets are inadequate in fiber, not providing the 20 to 30 grams daily that the average adult needs.

- Co-enzyme Q 10 has the ability to increase HDL and reduce platelet stickiness. It is an absolute must for people on statin drugs as well as a natural product I will speak of shortly, red yeast rice. An average daily dose is 100mg, although could be dependent upon other medications the individual is on that might be causing a further lowering of natural Co Q10 levels. CoQ10 also has shown to support blood sugar and insulin activity, as well as support healthy blood pressure.

Targeted Metabolic Support

Below you will find natural supplements that are beyond foundational, and can be found alone or in combination preparations to support certain risk factors and conditions of metabolic syndrome. If used in combination with medications, it is recommended to check with a knowledgeable physician or pharmacist as certain supplements can affect the metabolism and blood levels of medications, thus altering their activity. Also be aware that these ingredients might be found in other nutritional supplements, thus increasing the chances that someone might double up when not needed.

- Berberine- Berberine has many tremendous benefits across the spectrum of metabolic syndrome. Berberine has shown to lower LDL, lower total cholesterol, lower triglycerides, blood sugar and insulin, and provide healthy blood pressure and weight management.

- Niacin- Niacin comes with many healthy lipid benefits of decreasing total cholesterol and LDL, increases HDL, decreases triglycerides, and lower Lipoprotein A.

- Red Yeast Rice- Red Yeast Rice has the broad benefits of raising HDL, lowering LDL, lowering total cholesterol, and lowering triglycerides. It is recommend taking additional Co-Q10 and only sourcing a pharmaceutical grade product. Many different Co-Q10 products have shown to be riddled with pesticides and other toxins such as the mycotoxin citrinin. If someone has liver disease, like a statin drug, they should avoid this product.

- Plant Sterolins- Plant sterolins are a great addition for cholesterol management. I have seen tremendous benefits in these knocking down LDL, avoiding possible liver tie ups and even CoQ10 depletions that are often seen with the statin family of medications.

- Nattokinase- An ancient nutrient through food sources in Japan. This amazing nutrient that has shown to actually dissolve clots – thus one must be careful and let their doctor know if they are on blood thinning medications. Other benefits found are that it can lower cholesterol, improve blood pressure, improve circulation and even support bone density.

- Garlic- Garlic has shown many benefits such as lowering blood pressure, decreasing homocysteine as well as decreasing the clot promoting substance, fibrinogen. There are many different formulations of garlic on the market, so if you are looking for a particular benefit, make sure you go with a formula which has the research to back it up.

- Alpha Lipoic Acid - Increases insulin receptor sensitivity and efficacy leading to a decrease insulin resistance, which also leads it to be used in many weight loss programs.

- Chromium- Facilitates insulin and increases the uptake of glucose from the blood stream which leads to a decrease in excessive insulin production. Stimulates metabolism, and can decrease cholesterol, triglycerides and carbohydrate cravings.

- Vanadium- Has insulin like activity and can help to decrease blood sugar levels.

- Gymnea Sylvestre- Decreases blood sugar by stimulating release of insulin stores, and increases the activity of enzymes to utilize glucose.

- Bitter Melon- Enhances the body's ability to regulate blood sugar. Bitter Melon is believed to contain molecules that exert insulin like activity.

Metabolic Syndrome Checklist

1. Diet is first and foremost. Most of this metabolic mess we are in is a result to what has become the Standard American Diet (SAD). Refer back to earlier in this chapter where I provided the backbone for a proven, healthy metabolic diet; basically a Mediterranean or even a Paleo style diet.

2. Relaxation Techniques. This plays an enormous role in issues of metabolic disease, especially blood pressure. Refer to Part III, where I cover tools such as meditation, emotional freedom technique (EFT), and others.

3. Drug induced nutrient depletions. There are a litany of nutrient depletions caused by medications to treat the metabolic spectrum, from blood pressure, lipids and diabetes. Add to this the fact that most diets that lead to metabolic disorders are nutritionally empty, thus the need for healthy foundational nutrition while balancing off the imbalances.

4. Supplements. Incorporating a combination of foundational nutrition as well as targeted supplements can serve someone very well. Here are some general recommendations for some common problems to help guide your way. As always, check with your primary care practitioner.

   - Foundational Supplementation- Quality multivitamin and mineral complex and Essential Fatty Acids (ex- Fish Oil)

- High Lipids (Cholesterol and Triglycerides), High Insulin and/or Blood Sugar- Metabolic Extra from Pure Encapsulations, which contains berberine, alpha lipoic acid, chromium and resveratrol.

- High Lipids (Cholesterol and Triglycerides), Normal Insulin and/or Blood Sugar- Metabolic Extra from Pure Encapsulations or Berberine 500 from Thorne.

- High Lipids (Cholesterol and Triglycerides), Low Blood Sugar Problems- phytosterol product such as CholestePure or CholestePure Plus from Pure Encapsulations.

- High Triglycerides Only- Chromium such as Chromium GTF 600 from Pure Encapsulations, or Metabolic Extra from Pure Encapsulations.

- High Blood Sugar Insulin, Normal Lipid Levels- Glucofunction from Pure Encapsulations which contains ingredients such as bitter melon, chromium, vanadium, gymnena sylvestre, biotin, alpha lipoic acid and cinnamon.

- High Blood Pressure- Ensure adequate dose of magnesium (minimum of 300 mg daily), avoid in kidney disease until speaking to doctor. I have found good results additionally in Metagenics Vasotensin, or Pure Encapsulations Vascular Relax BP.

5. Exercise- Exercise plays a very big role in metabolic health. The important thing is to dial in the appropriate exercise routine for your needs. Check with your health care practitioner to find out what exercise program would be best for you.

See also; Sleep, Thyroid, and Stress, and Hormonal health and support.

Check out *www.wholepharmacy.com* for some of our favorite products containing many of the supplements mentioned above.

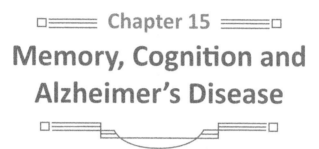

Chapter 15

Memory, Cognition and Alzheimer's Disease

From problems with memory to Alzheimer's disease; it seems that we are a nation in cognitive decline; and with the aging Baby Boomers this is a problem that is slated to become much greater- a medical tsunami on the horizon.

I like to break issues with memory and forgetfulness down to 4 categories. (1) Culturally related memory decline- General forgetfulness and memory problems due to mismanaged stress, depression, hypothyroidism, infections and diet which can happen at any age. (2) Age-related memory impairment (AMI) is the decline in various memory abilities and cognitive tasks associated with normal aging. (3) Mild Cognitive Impairment (MCI) is a condition in which people face memory problems more often than that of the average person their age.

Symptoms often include misplacing items, forgetting events or appointments, and having trouble thinking of desired words. MCI has been recognized as the transitional state that exists between age-related memory decline and Alzheimer's disease, and recent research suggests that it might be a mild form of Alzheimer's disease in itself. (4) Neurodegenerative conditions related to dementia and Alzheimer's disease.

Culturally Related Memory Decline

Stress

Stress works on many levels in affecting memory. We are designed to adapt to stress in a way that when stress is upon us, we respond, and then the stress goes away and we have a time of renewal and repair. The problem is that in our society and culture it seems stress never goes away, or people do not impart practical relaxation techniques and natural supplements to help the body adapt to the challenges of stress. In a typical hormonal response from the adrenal glands, when stress is upon us, cortisol rises, this is for protection of the body as we addressed in the chapter on stress. Optimally, when the stress is over, cortisol returns to normal. However in issues of chronic or mismanaged stress, this does not happen, cortisol levels stay high and your brain becomes a target. When exposed to high levels of cortisol the brain can actually be prevented from taking up the glucose needed for healthy brain function, the elevated and excess cortisol exposure can also slow your nerve impulse transmission as well which is critical in how the cells communicated. Cortisol will also take target at the hippocampus, the part of the brain that helps you sort and store your memories. Studies have shown in Alzheimer's patients that the size of their hippocampus is considerably reduced in size and activity.

Lack of Sleep

Speaking of stress, trouble sleeping is an epidemic in our society. Inadequate sleep has been linked to increase risk for diabetes, stroke, weight gain, impaired immune system, and you guessed it, memory loss. A recent report has tied regular good night's rest with living a long and healthier life.

This requirement of sleep for a long and healthy life is alarming since it is reported that only 38% of Baby Boomer's actually get a consistent, good night's rest. Part of the biology of a patient is what is known as beta amyloid plaques, and it has been shown that the growth of the amyloid actually slows down with adequate rest.

Thyroid

Hypothyroidism can lead to challenges with memory. If you remember in the section about thyroid we talked about how someone can be hypothyroid and not be assessed and treated adequately for reasons of inadequate testing and assessment. This is why it is so important to have a complete thyroid panel done which exceeds the common tests of T4 (levothyroxine) and TSH (thyroid stimulating hormone), and includes testing T3 (liothyronine), Thyroid antibodies, and reverse T3.

Depression

Depression can be a side-effect of hypothyroidism and stress. Depression itself can lead to memory problems, and so can hypothyroidism and stress, so as you can see these can be confounding factors. Thus reveals the importance for a holistic view on one's health, and not just treating the symptoms which in fact could lead to other problems. As you will see, depression and hypothyroidism are also risk factors to the advancement of Alzheimer's disease.

Gluten Intolerance

Estimates are that 1 in 10 people are intolerant to the protein gluten which is found in many grain based food products. Some estimates go even higher considering the rise in gluten in our food sources over the last decade or so, and many people go undiagnosed. One of the symptoms someone may have to a gluten reaction is memory problems and foggy thinking.

Infections

Yeast is a major culprit to memory problems, very much similar to someone reaction to gluten. It is because of this why it is important to dig deeper to identify what the individuals underlying problem might really be. Other infections such as viruses have shown to increase free radical activity, another common denominator in destruction of brain cells leading to dementia.

Hormonal Imbalance

Our society is becoming hormonally exhausted at an earlier age. Aside from the relationship of cortisol and stress and the effects on memory, steroid hormones such as estrogen and testosterone play important roles in maintaining a healthy memory, thus warrant a balanced assessment and treatment of bio-identical hormones if needed.

Sugar

Sugar and insulin resistance have major implications in Alzheimer's disease, and increased sugar through diet as well as unbalanced blood sugar levels can play a significant role in problems with memory. Remember how we spoke about the hippocampus and how cortisol will take aim and damage it as a result of mismanaged stress? Research shows that elevated blood sugar can result in reduced cerebral blood volume and blood flow in an area of the hippocampus leading to memory problems. Researchers said the effects can be seen even when levels of blood sugar, are only moderately elevated. Other studies in relation to sugar consumption in children have shown how sugar can negatively impact learning and retention.

Medications

There are numerous medications which can affect one's memory and cognition. The use of medications with anticholinergic activity increases the cumulative risk of cognitive impairment and mortality. These include certain allergy and sleep medications such as antihistamines, antidepressants and others. Statin drugs, the popular cholesterol lowering family of drugs has led to numerous cases of loss of short term memory, which should not be a major surprise since the brain utilizes 25% of the body's cholesterol. This is a class of drugs which I have already addressed, although I believe this memory and cognition element is going to be a growing concern as a major side-effect over the next few years. Sleeping pills such as Ambien® (zolpidem) and others have led to incidences of sleep walking and other dangerous activities also.

Supplements

General supplements to be included in a daily regimen which is preventative focused for healthy memory and cognition include: Alpha lipoic acid, CoQ10, EPA/DHA (fish oil), B Complex vitamins, selenium, Vitamin A, Vitamin C, Vitamin E, and anti-oxidants such as anthocyanin's.

Natural Supplements/Lifestyle for Culture Related Memory Impairment:

- Higher concentration DHA (Docosahexaenoic acid)
- Adaptogens- ex- American Ginseng and Rhodiola- Supports acute mental performance
- Bacopa- Supports learning, memory, mental performance, moderate stress.
- Phosphatidylserine- Supports memory, overall learning, recall, processing, in young and age related memory decline.
- Magnesium l-threonate- Supports cognitive function, learning, working memory, support health of the hippocampus
- Polyphenols (blueberry, strawberry, spinach) – Supports protection of brain neuropeptides involved with learning and memory as well as neurotransmitter activity and antioxidant protection.

Natural Supplements/Lifestyle for Age Related Memory Impairment:

- Gingko- Supports circulation and mental acuity.
- Vinpocitine- Supports mental performance and memory, healthy blood flow and glucose transport.
- Acetl-l-carnitine - Supports memory, emotional health, and cognitive function.

- Magnesium l-threonate- Supports cognitive function, learning, working memory, support health of the hippocampus (CogniMag®)
- Citicoline - Raises brain levels of acetylcholine and supports memory and mental performance. Some studies have shown that it's also able to reverse age-related changes in people with mild memory problems. As you will see below, medications for dementia and Alzheimer's are designed to prevent the destruction of acetylcholine.

Mild Cognitive Impairment

Mild cognitive impairment (MCI) is often the first recognized step into the conditions of dementia and Alzheimer's. MCI is recognized when someone begins to find it difficult to form new memories. Where this has been considered to a normal part of aging, recent studies have shown that MCI may not only be a marker for Alzheimer's, but may actually be a form of the disease.

Alzheimer's disease

Since Alzheimer's disease accounts for 50 to 80% of dementia cases and it is expected to grow so dramatically, we are going to focus the rest of this conversation on Alzheimer's disease.

Alzheimer's disease (AD) can be considered a medical tsunami building up to swamp and strain our health care system on many levels. Alzheimer's disease is already one of the most costly diseases in the world and recent reports are estimating that the number of people in the United States with AD will almost triple by 2050, from about 5 million now to 13.8 million.

This dramatic increase is largely due to the aging baby boomers, those born between 1946 and 1964. AD currently affects 1 in 8 people over age 65, and half of people over 85.

Alzheimer's disease is an incurable, progressive, neurodegenerative disease characterized by a loss of memory, cognition, affects personality and behavior eventually leading to even routine tasks such as dressing and bathing impossible, leaving these patients completely dependent on others for care.

Alzheimer's disease is highly associated with the development of amyloid plaques in the brain, similar in many ways to the plaques that clog artery walls and eventually lead to heart attacks. These plaques are known as beta-amyloid, or Amyloid beta (Aβ). Aβ is a group of amino acids that form from the Amyloid precursor protein (APP). Aβ is the main component of deposits found in the brains of patients with Alzheimer's disease.

There is no single test that can show whether a person has Alzheimer's. Diagnosing Alzheimer's requires a thorough medical evaluation, including: a thorough medical history and symptom assessment, a physical and neurological exam, and tests such as blood tests and brain imaging to either rule out other causes of dementia-like symptoms, or to identify biological formations such as the beta amyloid plaques mentioned above.

The social, financial and health related impacts are extensive. With the rising number of cases, the financial impacts of caring for patients with Alzheimer's and other forms of dementia are expected to increase 500% by 2050, reaching $1.1 trillion. The Alzheimer's Association says patients with Alzheimer's and other forms of dementia will spend three times more on health care than patients with other types of illnesses.

Alzheimer's presents a major time and financial burden on caregivers, families and friends. In 2011, 15.2 million family and friends provided 17.4 billion hours of unpaid care to those with Alzheimer's and other dementias- care valued at $210.5 billion. According to a 2011 study shown that women who take time off or quit work to care for a loved one lose an average of $324,044 in lifetime wages, pension and Social Security benefits; for men, the average loss is $283,716. Three out of five people needing care are cared for at home, while almost 75% of home care is provided by family and friends.

In regards to health impact, those with Alzheimer's are three times more likely to face hospitalization and eight times more likely to need skilled nursing care, with one-fourth of all home care involves care for an Alzheimer's patient.

There a number of risk Factors for MCI and Alzheimer's disease, including; (1) family history - if someone's first-degree relative (mother, father, or sibling) has Alzheimer's, the chances are up to seven times greater that they may develop the disease, (2) APOe-4 gene - a person with two APOe-4 genes is at a higher risk of developing Alzheimer's disease, (3) depression, (4) hypothyroidism, (5) free radicals, (6) insulin resistance, metabolic syndrome and diabetes, and (7) head injury. The good news is that many risk factors can be controlled effectively by adopting correct lifestyle choices as we will cover shortly.

Heavy Metals, Aluminum and Alzheimer's Disease

Years ago it was discovered that there was a common occurrence in the brains of those who died of Alzheimer's disease, a significant amount of aluminum deposited in the brain tissue compared to others who did not die with the disease.

Many diseases we are dealing with are diseases as a result of our environment, inside and outside of the body, which relate to the bodies in ability to effectively deal with toxic load. Aluminum is one of the major challenges as it is found in water supplies, food sources, and vaccinations.

We will speak more about measures of cleansing and detoxification in Chapter 17, although for now, I just want you to recognize that this is of major concern for Alzheimer's while little is done through Western medicine to address it.

Free Radicals and Alzheimer's Disease

Free radicals have been linked to the main diseases of aging and generative disease, including heart disease, cancer, arthritis, and more, and you should not be surprised to find out that free radicals are also believed to be an important cause of Alzheimer's disease.

Free radicals are unstable substances in your body that attack your body's cells. Free radicals result naturally from the process of oxidation (respiration, digestive processes, etc.), although when you are exposed to high levels of pollutants, such as environmental toxins, cigarette smoke, or even many foods you eat, your production of free radicals increases and your body may fall victim to their damaging effects.

Antioxidants through food and supplements are the natural combatants to free radicals, although when free radicals win the battle it is known as oxidative stress. Studies have shown that Alzheimer's sufferers experience a greater degree of oxidative stress and damage in their brains and to their brain neurons than those without the disease. The result is accelerated brain aging and brain cell death.

Other contributing factors to higher levels of free radicals and/or their resulting oxidative stresses on your brain may include:

- Inflammation
- Head trauma
- Heavy metals
- Viral infections
- Pesticides
- Electromagnetic fields
- Having the Apo-E4 gene
- Melatonin deficiency
- Elevated homocysteine
- High fat diet
- Depression
- Vitamin B12 deficiency
- Folic acid deficiency
- Hormone imbalances

- Lack of mental stimulation
- Lack of physical exercise

As far as supplementation, the polyphenol family of antioxidants has shown tremendous benefits from improvement of memory, free radical protection, and even in influencing healthy gene expression. Polyphenols from berries such as blueberries and strawberries, as well as spinach have been used in novel phytomemory blends, such as PS Plus by Pure Encapsulations, which is often one of my foremost recommendations in the area of healthy cognitive function.

The Relationships between Diabetes and Alzheimer's disease

Alzheimer's disease is now being linked to insulin resistance and diabetes in what is being called Type III Diabetes, also referred to as Brain Diabetes. This dangerous hybrid form of Diabetes was confirmed during a study which took place at Brown University's Medical School. That study showed for the first time exactly how the brain produces and uses insulin, which very closely mirrors the way that the pancreas makes it. Insulin has proven to be critical for memory, and too little, or what is called "insulin resistance" has now been implicated in Alzheimer's disease and other dementia related disorders.

There is also a relationship between the protein plaques found in Alzheimer's disease. The way the brain makes insulin can result in the formation of this plaque which resembles plaque in cardiac arteries found in Type 1 and Type 2 diabetes patients. However, the attack of the brain's functions is the result with *Type 3 Diabetes,* and memory loss and improper memory creation and formation are the result.

Those who suffer from Alzheimer's disease and *Type 3 Diabetes* tend to have much lower levels of insulin, or are insulin-resistant. Researchers discovered that memory creation fails when insulin is in short supply because insulin is good at warding off dangerous amyloid beta-derived diffusible ligands (ADDLs). These bad guys destroy receptors in your brain when insulin is not around to shield them, and they cannot connect the synapses, and thus also can't form memories.

Alzheimer's and Cardiovascular Disease

Hippocrates stated some 2,500 years ago, "whatever is good for the heart is probably good for the brain," and this is true in so many ways; from development of plaques, to similar dietary, preventative and treatment options in both disease states. Take for instance homocysteine. Elevated homocysteine is a risk factor for heart disease (we talked about this in the section on metabolic syndrome). Elevated homocysteine can also be a reason for increased free radical attack in the body, which in itself can lead to Alzheimer's disease. So as you can see, by reducing a risk factor for heart disease such as homocysteine, you are also reducing a major risk factor for Alzheimer's disease.

5 Keys to Alzheimer's Prevention, Preparation and Slowing Progression

There is no known cure for Alzheimer's and other related disorders of dementia; although there are many things we can do as far as prevention minded strategies and to slow the progression of the disease. The information here can be utilized for any issue of cognitive decline or form of dementia, and it is best to approach this in a holistic mindset, not just focusing on one of the keys, but most or all of them.

There are 5 keys that work synergistically in preventing the onset as well as slowing the progression of cognitive decline, dementia and Alzheimer's.

Key #1: Diet

The Back Bone To A Healthy Diet: Mediterranean / Paleo style diet

We talked about the similarities in treating and preventing conditions of Alzheimer's and heart disease, and as one might expect, they have similar recommended diets. In fact, a healthy diet is no mystery; a general healthy diet share will share some very common factors and can provide tremendous benefits in many disease states.

Population studies have shown that people more than 85 years old who eat fish have a 40 percent smaller risk of developing Alzheimer's. Other research has shown that the brains of Alzheimer's patients have 30 percent less DHA than the brains of healthy individuals. In data from the landmark Framingham Heart Study, those patients who had lower levels of long-chain Omega-3 fatty acids in their blood had a 67 percent greater likelihood of developing Alzheimer's. In fact, supplementation with DHA seems to improve the cognitive function of Alzheimer's patients, according to one intervention study.

Research is finding that olive oil helps shuttle the abnormal amyloid proteins out of the brain in a new study that appears in the journal ACS Chemical Neuroscience. Amal Kaddoumi and colleagues note that AD affects about 30 million people worldwide, but the prevalence is lower in Mediterranean countries. Scientists once attributed it to the high concentration of healthful monounsaturated fats in olive oil--consumed in large amounts in the Mediterranean diet. Newer research suggested that the actual protective agent might be a substance called oleocanthal, which has effects that protect nerve cells from the kind of damage that occurs in AD. Kaddoumi's team sought evidence on whether oleocanthal helps decrease the accumulation of beta-amyloid in the brain, believed to be the culprit in AD.

They describe tracking the effects of oleocanthal in the brains and cultured brain cells of laboratory mice used as stand-ins for humans in such research. In both instances, oleocanthal showed a consistent pattern in which it boosted production of two proteins and key enzymes believed to be critical in removing beta amyloid from the brain. "Extra-virgin olive oil-derived oleocanthal associated with the consumption of Mediterranean diet has the potential to reduce the risk of AD or related neurodegenerative dementias," the report concludes.

Additionally, research has shown that Alzheimer's disease might be related to toxicity, thus reduction of excitotoxins such as aspartame and MSG, heavy metals in foods and environment, processed foods, artificial flavorings and sweeteners in one's food is also recommended. Let's just get back to eating real food.

Key #2: Supplements

As far as memory, cognitive decline and neurodegenerative disease such as Alzheimer's, nutritional supplementations can play a major role. From supplements to support healthy cognitive function to others which have shown to slow the progression of biological disease states, here are some of our favorites.

When talking about Alzheimer's disease, the progression and biology, let's take a look at some of the most promising research on natural supplementation which will include; Curcumin, Vitamin D3, Resveratrol, Berberine , Green Tea, and the antioxidant family known as anthocyanin's.

Studies have shown that the combination of curcumin and vitamin D3 can help reduce Alzheimer's plaques through immunomodulation and regulation. Curcumin by itself has been found to accelerate nerve fiber formation by reducing the amount of oligomers, which are thought to be harmful to the nerve cells and responsible for the formation of the amyloid, which is linked to Alzheimer's plaques. It is important to point out that through food, curcumin has a very low bioavailability, and thus we recommend using a high bioavailable nutritional supplement source.

Resveratrol has shown to neutralize the free radicals created from the amyloid and Alzheimer's plaques, as well as its ability to neutralize free radicals at the inception of the process, thus another critical step in the defense against Alzheimer's disease.

Berberine has shown tremendous benefits in metabolic support including; lowering blood sugar, low density lipoprotein (LDL), and triglycerides. And remember how we spoke about Alzheimer's being called type III diabetes? Well the following benefits of berberine should not surprise you, and would show berberine to be critical in Alzheimer's prevention especially in someone with metabolic syndrome or diabetes.

Recent findings show that berberine prevents neuronal damage due to ischemia or oxidative stress, and it has been reported that berberine reduces amyloid-beta peptide (AP) levels by modulating APP processing. The accumulation of amyloid-beta peptide (AP) derived from amyloid precursor protein (APP) is a triggering event leading to the pathological cascade of Alzheimer's disease (AD); therefore the inhibition of AP production should be a rational therapeutic strategy in the prevention and treatment of AD.

Green tea has long been hailed as a cardio-protective beverage due to its ability to lower levels of oxidized LDL cholesterol, an established heart disease risk factor. It has also been shown to promote brain health because the active compound, EGCG (Epigallocatechin gallate) freely crosses the blood-brain barrier to provide antioxidant support and lower damaging levels of brain inflammation.

Researchers from Japan reporting in the *American Journal of Clinical Nutrition* demonstrate that regular green tea consumption lowers the risk of developing functional disabilities that lead to problems with daily chores and activities, such as bathing or dressing. Drinking up to five cups of green tea each day can lower the risk of developing functional disabilities as we age by nearly one half.

The researchers noted that those consuming five or more cups of green tea each day also ate more fruit and vegetables, consumed more fish, were less likely to smoke, had fewer strokes or heart attacks, and tended to have a higher level of education. Improved dietary and lifestyle considerations are synergistic factors that compliment green tea consumption and likely contribute to the positive results in this study.

Health-minded individuals already follow strict dietary principles to maintain brain health and functional abilities. Drinking 5 or more cups of green tea each day are shown to boost the healthy benefits associated with proper nutrition and lifestyle. Supplements with concentrated EGCG are a great alternative for those not looking to consume 5 cups of green tea daily, plus are standardized for quality control.

Very recent and exciting research has shown that green tea can actually decrease the production of the amyloid plaques prevalent in Alzheimer's patients. Researchers at the University of Michigan have found a new potential benefit of a molecule in green tea: preventing the mis-folding of specific proteins in the brain. The aggregation of these proteins, called metal-associated amyloids, is associated with Alzheimer's disease and other neurodegenerative conditions.

In this study, researchers used green tea extract to control the generation of metal-associated amyloid-β aggregates associated with Alzheimer's disease in the lab. They found that the specific molecule in green tea, epigallocatechin-3-gallate, also known as EGCG, prevented aggregate formation and broke down existing aggregate structures in the proteins that contained metals -- specifically copper, iron and zinc.

Antioxidants such as polyphenols are part of the flavonoid family. Plants rich in these antioxidants include blueberry, cranberry, bilberry, black raspberry, red raspberry, blackberry, blackcurrant, cherry, and Concord grape. A growing body of evidence suggests these antioxidants may possess neuro-protective and anti-inflammatory activities.

A study in the British Journal of Nutrition shown that study participants who consumed 2 cups each day of grape juice, greatly improved their learning and recall. This study has been reproduced with other sources rich in anthocyanin activity such as blueberry juice as well.

So as you can see, incorporating some critical nutrients via food and supplements can have a wide range of benefits in regards to prevention or reducing the advancement of Alzheimer's disease.

As far as supplements, from a preventative minded approach, my favorites are Rescue SR from Pure which contains curcumin and resveratrol, optimized vitamin D levels and to supplement with a quality D3 if needed, and PS Plus, which contains phosphatidylserine along with a polyphenol memory blend (this is also good for issues of age related memory disorders.)

Key #3: Stress Relieving Techniques and Management

Balancing and helping your body and mind to adapt to daily stress is a critical part of any Alzheimer prevention strategy. We have talked about the negative effects of stress on our overall health, as well as brain and memory health. Stress relieving techniques include meditation, breathing techniques, guided imagery and visualization, hypnosis, and even moving meditations combined with exercise such as yoga and qigong.

Meditation itself has shown tremendous benefits in regards to allowing the body to adapt to stress, thus reducing the impact that stress has on memory and cognition. Let's first look at what exactly happens in regards to our body's reaction to stress when we meditate. Meditation not only will help you feel more relaxed, meditation lowers cortisol, reduces the beta wave stimulation and shifts and begins to emit alpha waves and sometimes even the deeper delta waves.

The Alzheimer's research and prevention foundation (ARPF) has investigated and found great success in specific meditation known as Kirtan Kriya. ARPF reports that this practice holds tremendous potential to bolster the effects of medication and other strategies used to slow or prevent Alzheimer's disease. The foundation believes it may even hold the potential to reverse memory loss.

Kirtan Kriya (pron. Keertun Kreea) is a type of meditation from the Kundalini yoga tradition, which has been practiced for thousands of years. This meditation is sometimes called a singing exercise, as it involves singing the sounds, *Saa Taa Naa Maa* along with repetitive finger movements, or *mudras*. This non-religious practice can be adapted to several lengths, but practicing it for just 12 minutes a day has been shown to reduce stress levels and increase activity in areas of the brain that are central to memory.

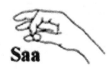 **Saa** 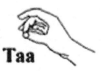 **Taa** 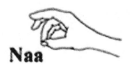 **Naa** 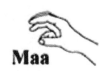 **Maa**

You can find more out about the Kirtan Kriya at the ARPF website where they present a multitude of studies, www.alzheimersprevention.org/research.htm, although let me share with you one of the findings in a study published in the International Journal of Geriatric Psychiatry which shows tremendous benefits for this form of meditation which incorporates active mental meditation and "singing" and not just relaxation.

"A pilot study of yogic meditation for family dementia caregivers with depressive symptoms: Effects on mental health, cognition, and telomerase activity."

In a groundbreaking study completed in January 2011, and published in the International Journal of Geriatric Psychiatry, in collaboration with UCLA, we investigated the effects of meditation in caregivers of people with dementia. Results indicate that, compared to study participants who listened to relaxation tapes daily for eight weeks, those who practiced Kirtan Kriya improved significantly in measures of perceived support, physical suffering, energy, emotional well-being, cognitive tests of memory and executive function. Beyond that, this study revealed that Kirtan Kriya increased telomerase, an exquisite bio marker of health and longevity. In this study, we showed that mood, spirituality, and well-being; all markers of improved memory health and longevity, can be increased by Kirtan Kriya in only 12 minutes a day for 12 weeks.

Key #4: Exercise

Movement is the key, physical and metal movement and there have been numerous studies that shown how both physical and mental exercises can benefit memory as well as support preventative measures in Alzheimer's disease. In fact studies have shown that aerobic exercise as little as 3 times a week for 6 months resulted in the expansion of gray matter in the brain, the area of retaining memory and focus. Other studies have shown regular exercise to reverse age related shrinkage of the brain.

Regular exercise can reduce your risk for developing Alzheimer's disease by up to 50%, and most experts will agree that an overall active lifestyle is the key to optimum brain and body health. As far as physical exercise research shows that you should do the equivalent of walking a minimum of

20 minutes three times a week, although incorporating different types of exercise such as dancing, swimming, tennis, can be of additional benefit. The key is to find something you enjoy and have fun with it.

A recent study published in the Annals of Internal Medicine that suggests that staying fit in your mid-life years might help forestall dementia down the road. Researchers looked at a cohort of just under 20,000 adults who had taken treadmill fitness tests at a health clinic at some time before they turned 65; they then used Medicare records to track the adults' incidence of dementia over the ensuing years. (The average subject was followed for 24 years, post-test.) Those who scored in the top quintile for fitness on the treadmill test were 36% less likely to suffer from dementia than those in the bottom quintile.

Combining mental stimulation with exercise shows even greater benefit. I mentioned above the benefits of dance as an aerobic exercise, and numerous studies point to the benefits of dancing and memory. One particular study stands out in that it shown much more benefit when participants continue learning new dances, they progress better and retain working memory better.

With exercise comes the benefit of "preparation" in the case of Alzheimer's disease. Where I don't want to look at preparation as a self-fulfilling prophecy, more of a "ignorance is no longer bliss," if in fact someone was to go down the path of AD, coming to the table with strength and balance would be a tremendous benefit.

Mental Exercise

Even if it's not with physical exercise, mental exercise has shown tremendous benefits in memory and cognitive support. Neurologists report that mental exercise can reduce your chance of developing Alzheimer's disease by up to 70%.

If you look at the rates of cognitive decline and Alzheimer's many developed countries have the highest number of cases. Much of this might be due to the fact that if you don't use it, you lose it. One should exercise their brain cells regularly or else he/she will lose them for good. Developed nations provide almost everything needed for people to stay static; remote controls, packaged foods, fast food delivered, thus their brain cells aren't exercising. This causes these cells to die bit by bit. Underdeveloped nations do not have the problem with people at any age staying static.

So you just have to challenge your brain with new and novel tasks such as reading about new topics of information (learning), writing (journaling is a great exercise), board games, crossword puzzles, sudoku, learning new language's, etc.

In Mary Lou Henners book, *Total Memory Make Over*, she shares the acronym, APR which stands for Anticipation, Participation, and Recollection. This is essentially suggesting staying present, mindful, and conscious every day. I shudder to think what people are doing to their brain capacity as they walk around in a haze focusing in on their 'smart' phones, frying their brains, most likely making themselves dumber.

In the formula of APR, these are three parts to every event, and focusing on these three will help to exercise your brain.

Ask yourself:

What am I anticipating today?

What am I in the middle of, what am I participating in?

What can I be recollecting from today?

Another great resource for this is online, Lumosity, *http://www.lumosity.com/*. This uses the science of neuroplasticity in the form of games, to help train the brain in a healthier direction.

Key #5: Hormones and Medications

Hormone replacement therapy plays a very big role in memory retention and cognitive behavior. Our hormones are our great communicators, and if hormonal function is depleted, communication and memory can falter. This is why I recommend a proper assessment of thyroid, adrenal health, and sex steroid hormones, from a qualified practitioner, experienced in bio identical hormonal balance.

Bio-identical hormones are always a hot topic, often conventional minded practitioners speaking against them for "lack of evidence based results" which is largely untrue. There is a growing library of strong clinical support for the proper balance and replacement of bio-identical hormones in your body. One of the best resources for this would be to contact a compounding pharmacy to find a practitioner who is experienced and qualified in this area of medicine.

Conventional pharmaceutical therapy due have their place in a holistic model of Alzheimer's treatment. If going to a conventional only practitioner these are often the only form of treatment which will be offered, which I believe leaves the patient at a disadvantage of not having all the tools at their service which they could use.

Below are the most common medications currently being prescribed for the treatment of Alzheimer's, and as you will see have generally different degrees of benefits.

For more information, speak to your pharmacist or physician and I don't recommend these to be stand-alone therapy, optimally they will be used with some of the other keys mentioned above.

Aricept (donepezil): Aricept is moderately effective in improving short-term memory in patients with early Alzheimer's. Aricept works by stopping a specific enzyme from breaking down acetylcholine in the brain, which can help improve memory, attention, reason, language, and the ability to perform simple tasks.

Exelon (rivastigmine): Exelon has shown to be slightly more effective than Aricept at slowing the rate of decline in a patient with Alzheimer's because in its effort to prevent the breakdown of acetylcholine in the brain, it blocks two chemical pathways and not just one.

Namenda (memantine): Memantine has shown a modest effect in alleviating some of the symptoms for people suffering with advanced Alzheimer's disease. Namenda works differently than the other two by blocking a brain chemical called glutamate, which has been implicated in brain cell death. Remember how we said that cortisol takes aim at the hippocampus and memory? Cortisol also disrupts glutamate function inside the brain.

This disruption causes many free radicals to form inside your brain cell, thus lead to cell death. Namenda is believed to reverse this disruption, although this shows the benefits to address the cortisol issue earlier in life for optimal brain health.

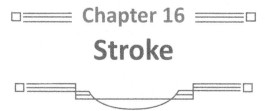

Chapter 16

Stroke

According to the National Stroke Association, stroke is the fourth leading cause of death and the leading cause of adult disability in the United States. It should come as no surprise considering that many of the risk factors and preventative measures for strokes fall in line with most of what we spoke about in metabolic syndrome and brain, memory, cognition and Alzheimer's disease. From diet, to supplements, to lifestyle choices including exercise and relaxation techniques, there are numerous similarities in risk factors and preventative measures.

A stroke, also referred to as a cerebral vascular accident, occurs when blood supply to the brain is interrupted and the brain is deprived of oxygen, and brain damage can ensue.

Different Kinds of Strokes:

Ischemic- Most common (87% of cases), a blood vessel s blocked to the brain.

Embolic- begins elsewhere in body and travels to brain.

Thrombotic- forms in an artery in the brain.

Hemorrhagic- An artery in brain leaks or bursts. Brain damage can happen within minutes. Quick treatment is a must to limit damage and increase chance of full recovery.

Transient Ischemic Attack (TIA) - This should be taking as a warning for a future stroke. A vessel becomes blocked for a short period of time, few minutes to 24 hours

Aneurism- A week spot develops in the wall of an artery, results in ballooning, if gets bigger, becomes even weaker and can burst and leak blood

General stroke symptoms include:

- Sudden numbness or weakness in face, arms or legs
- Sudden confusion, trouble speaking, or understanding
- Sudden trouble seeing in one or both eyes
- Sudden trouble walking, dizziness, loss of balance or coordination
- Sudden severe headache with no known cause

Five Stroke Prevention and Preparative Minded Strategies

According to the National Stroke Association, up to 80 percent of strokes are preventable. When I mention preparing for a stroke, this is not to suggest a self-fulfilling prophecy, but instead to have the body prepared to be as healthy as possible to be able to respond and recover in the best possible way. Below are 5 strategies and factors to arm yourself to reduce your chances of a stroke, and if in fact one was to occur, to prepare the body for the best possible way to respond and repair.

You will see I list medications as a factor, more so from a treatment after the fact mode. Our system of emergency medicine has done wonderful things to respond to stroke victims, although it is critical to get treatment as soon as possible. As far as medications for maintenance treatment after a stroke, or even used as a preventative, depending on the medication, one must be very careful for interactions with other medications and even nutrients, thus always clear your supplements and other medications with your physician.

1. Recognize and Address Risk Factors

- **High Blood Pressure**- If left untreated, hypertension can lead to stroke, cardiovascular disease as well as a wide variety of other life-threatening conditions, such as kidney damage and congestive heart failure.

- **Total Cholesterol, LDL Cholesterol, HDL Cholesterol, and VLDL Cholesterol** – A standard cholesterol profile usually consists of measuring Total Cholesterol, LDL Cholesterol and HDL Cholesterol. High levels of total cholesterol, LDL cholesterol and low levels of HDL have consistently been associated with risk of cardiovascular disease- it's about balance. VLDL (Very-low-density lipoprotein) cholesterol is a type of lipoprotein which contains the highest amount of triglyceride. Having a high VLDL level means you may have an increased risk of coronary artery disease, which can lead to a heart attack, high blood pressure or stroke.

- **Triglycerides**- Triglycerides are the form that fat takes when it is being stored for energy in your body. Triglycerides, liked cholesterol, are vital for human life but unhealthy if at too high a level.

- **Homocysteine**- Amino acid which promotes free radical production, can lead to elevated triglycerides, elevated cholesterol, and has a direct relationship to stroke, cardiovascular and pulmonary vascular disease.

- **C-Reactive Protein** - A protein that is found in the blood. Its levels become elevated when the body detects an infection or need for inflammation. Elevated levels may also indicate future problems including cardiovascular disease and atherosclerosis.

- **Diabetes and Insulin Resistance**- Several studies have proven that insulin resistance can cause increases in blood pressure which is already a known risk factor. Elevated levels of insulin can cause atherosclerosis, and research Researchers found that pre-diabetes based on the 1997 American Diabetes Association (ADA) definition of 110 to 125 mg/dl carried a 21% higher chance of stroke.

- **Smoking**- Smoking is a known risk factor for stroke, thus prudent to quit.

- **Excessive Alcohol Consumption** – Where a drink can show some benefits in stroke prevention, it is important to avoid excessive consumption since it can increase stroke risks.

- **Stress**- The more stressed you are, the greater your risk for stroke. One study found that for every notch lower a person scored on their well-being scale, their risk of stroke increased by 11 percent.

- **Obesity**- Obesity is a risk factor for stroke and is often linked to other risk factors such as insulin resistance, diabetes, and cardiovascular disease.

- **Arteriosclerosis**- Arteriosclerosis is a build-up of plaque in the arteries which is composed of calcium, cellular waste, fibrinogen, fat, and cholesterol, which can directly lead to blockage of arteries.

- **Free Radicals**- Free radicals are risk factors for strokes to happen and are also a result of the stroke thus causing more cellular damage.

- **Medications**- NSAID's, synthetic estrogens in birth control pills and hormonal therapy, Avandia, Evista.

- **Atrial Fibrillation (A Fib)** – Atrial fibrillation is an irregular heartbeat which can result in a pooling of blood within the arteries that can build into a blockage.

2. Diet- Paleo/Mediterranean

   Goal of a diet is to protect the blood vessels, oxygenate the tissues, and fight damaging free radicals

   - Lots of fresh vegetables, fruits, whole grains and lean protein

   - Unprocessed, and natural food choices

   - Avoid: Diet sodas, trans-fats, smoked and processed meats (nitrites ex-sodium nitrite damages blood vessels,) MSG, Aspartame, preservatives, artificial flavorings and colors, GMO's.

   - Lycopene rich foods (tomatoes, watermelon, apricots, guava, papaya, pink grapefruit) - One study shown lycopene reduced stroke risk by 55 % in men.

3. Nutrition and Supplements

   Vitamin D- The benefits of healthy vitamin D levels continue to mount. Low vitamin D levels have been associated with arterial stiffness. One study found that people who got less than the midpoint level of sun exposure were at a 60 percent increased risk for stroke, while a Finland study found that the lowest vitamin D levels were twice as likely to get a stroke as people with highest vitamin D levels.

   Vitamin K2- D and K2 work synergistically to inhibit arterial calcification, component of plaques and arteriosclerosis.

   B Vitamins (B6, B12, Folic Acid) - Reduce homocysteine.

   CoQ10- Antioxidant, neuroprotection, cardiovascular homeostasis, membrane stabilizer. Keep in mind that many medications to lower cholesterol and blood pressure, and even blood sugar can deplete CoQ10.

Magnesium- Healthy vascular relaxation, decreases blood vessel constriction, relaxes electrical impulses and encourages calmness, maintains the normal rhythm of your heart, increases HDL (good) cholesterol. It is estimated that 50% of North Americans are deficient in magnesium and those deficient have double the risk of a cardiovascular event. Magnesium is also a nutrient which is commonly depleted by medication therapy.

EPA/DHA- Helps lower lipid and blood sugar risk factors including inflammation.

Nattokinase- An ancient nutrient through food sources in Japan. This amazing nutrient that has shown to actually dissolve clots by decreasing fibrin, an active part of arterial plaque build-up – thus one must be careful and let their doctor know if they are on blood thinning medications. Other benefits found are that it can lower cholesterol, improve blood pressure, improve circulation and even support bone density.

Antioxidants- Provide free radical defense and more.

Polyphenol blends- Neuro and vascular protective- cranberry, blueberry, strawberry, spinach, turmeric via curcumin, resveratrol, green tea, and grape seed.

Resveratrol- Antioxidant activity, healthy platelet function.

Pomegranate- Antioxidant and vascular support.

Curcumin- Antioxidant support with other benefits including; healthy inflammatory balance, liver support, brain and cognitive support, protection against radiation, natural chemotherapeutic agent.

As far as supplements, from a preventative minded approach, my favorites are Quality EPA/DHA supplementation, Magnesium, Rescue SR from Pure which contains curcumin and resveratrol, optimized vitamin D levels and to supplement with a quality D3 if needed, and PS Plus, which contains phosphatidylserine along with a polyphenol memory blend (this is also good for issues of age related memory disorders and offers the neuro protective benefits.)

4. Medications

Cholesterol Lowering Drugs- Stain drugs are a common cholesterol lowering medication and can make platelets less likely to stick together leading to a clot, although studies have shown an increased chance of a second stroke in those who have had previous hemorrhagic based stroke. One study shown that in people who already have had a stroke related to bleeding in the brain, those who took statins had a 22 percent risk of a second stroke, those not on statins, a 14 percent.

Anticoagulants- Reduce risk of blood clots and prevent existing blood clots from getting bigger by thinning blood.

- Heparin
- Pradaxa- Used in cases of atrial fibrillation.
- Coumadin (warfarin) - Broad use anticoagulant must be carefully monitored.
- Xarelto- Used in cases of atrial fibrillation, deep vein thrombosis, pulmonary embolisms, knee or hip replacements.

Antiplatelet Medications- Prevents platelets from sticking together.

- Persantine (dypridamole)
- Aggrenox (aspirin and dypridamole)
- Ticlid (ticlodopine)
- Plavix (clopiderol)

Angiotensin II receptor Antagonists- Block and enzyme that triggers muscle contracting around the blood vessels, thus narrowing them, thus blood vessels can enlarge and blood pressure is reduced.

Antithrombotic- Aspirin

5. Relaxation techniques- The more stressed you are, the greater your risk for stroke. One study found that for every notch lower a person scored on their well-being scale, their risk of stroke increased by 11 percent.

Embrace relaxation techniques and strategies to support emotional health and stress such as: meditation, prayer, yoga, breathing techniques, tai chi, qigong, emotional freedom technique (EFT), etc. Additionally, have your adrenal health properly assessed, and refer to chapter 10 on stress.

As in all areas of disease and wellness, we like to look at a preventative mentality first, thus diet, lifestyle and supplements. Take a look at the medications such as the angiotension II receptor antagonists. As they are designed to prevent the contracting of muscles around the blood vessels, magnesium, with its relaxation properties offers a preventative minded approach, the same with the relaxation benefits of meditation, yoga and other disciplines. The same with the antiplatelet medications and the nutrient resveratrol as it has shown to promote healthy platelet activity.

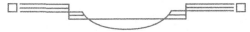

Chapter 17

Detoxification and Cleansing

Have you ever had fish as pets? Did your fish ever get sick? If so, what was the recommended treatment? Clean the fish tank, their environment, right? It's no different with you and me. The problem with our medical system is that when someone has a symptom, instead of clearing the pathways for healing such as is taught through natural systems of medicine, a prescription is prescribed. In many cases a prescription only quiets the symptoms and does not get to the root of the problem, and the problem will continue to build or will lead to other issues such as we have seen in the issue of the over-prescribing of antibiotics.

In addition, medications can actually further suppress the body's natural ability to heal; challenging detoxification systems such as the liver, kidneys and gallbladder, induce nutrient depletions which are needed for healing and optimal health and more.

Remember in the mind body section how I mentioned researchers such as Bruce Lipton PHD have proven that our health is the product of our environment; the thoughts we think, the foods we eat, and the exercise we do and don't do? Bruce Lipton has shared that in one of his experiment's, when you continue to change the environment that a cell culture lives in to allow it to be cleaner and more pure, the longer the cells will live.

So when we get sick, diagnosed with a disease, why does the medical system not address the environment in a multi-dimensional fashion? Remember, the outer layer of the cell is the cells equivalent to the brain, and as you damage the outer layer by the environment the cell is bathed in, the increase risk you have to damage the cell itself, thus usher in disease.

We live in a toxic environment, and regular cleanses should be part of our health maintenance program throughout the year as well as regularly consuming foods which aids us in this process. On a daily basis we are all exposed to toxins such as heavy metals, PCB' s, gasses, pesticides, xenoestrogens, excitotoxins, and more through avenues such as:

- Cleaning agents
- Fuel
- Cosmetics/Personal Care- deodorants and aluminum, skin care products, fluoride in tooth paste
- Building Materials
- Cigarettes, smoke and ash
- Carpet
- Furniture
- Toys
- Batteries/Car batteries

- Medications/Vaccines/Dental amalgams
- Putty (toys and industrial)
- Impure supplements
- Genetically modified seeds
- Plastics/packaging
- Lawns, gardens, farms, plants, golf courses
- Foods- non organic- herbicides
- Fish/mercury
- Cooking wear
- Pillows/mattresses/clothing
- Water/rain/snow
- Fabric softeners
- Radiation
- Tattoos
- Artificial sweeteners, food colors, food additives
- Low quality supplements

A Toxic Burden Can Lead To:

- Gastrointestinal disorders such as constipation, diarrhea, gas, IBS and other digestive problems
- Excess weight that seems impossible to get off
- Inflammation, arthritis, joint and muscle pains
- Fatigue and exhaustion
- Headaches, fuzzy thinking, decreased memory and concentration
- Difficulty sleeping and even behavioral issues such as feeling agitated, irritated, hyperactivity
- Hormonal imbalances

The ways the body may respond to toxins vary, depending on someone's constitutional make-up, genetics, and toxic load and ability to metabolize. This all can be affected by current medication and supplements which may influence their ability to metabolize toxins.

Almost every disease state can have an element tied to toxic overload, to one degree or another including: Chronic Fatigue, Fibromyalgia, Multiple Chemical Sensitivity (MCS), Alzheimer's, Parkinson's, ALS/Lou Gehrig's, Huntington's Disease, Thyroid and other hormonal imbalances, Autism Spectrum Disorders, Cardiovascular issues and more.

Studies have shown that the average American contains between 400 and 800 chemicals and heavy metals stored in their fat tissues. Leading experts agree that toxins play a role in almost everyone known illness, no one is immune. These estimates should not be surprising, considering an average day for an average American.

The body has a natural ability to detoxify through the liver/gallbladder, the large intestines and the kidneys as well as the lymphatic system, if we provide it the environment to do so. The problem is if these areas are compromised, the detox process gets hampered and one begins to either recycle their toxins and/or begins to deposit these toxins into fat tissues, glands and organs.

When the EPA (Environmental Protection Agency) and other agencies decide the safety levels of toxins, they look at each toxins impact as a single entity, but do not look at the accumulative issue of multiple toxins all at once challenging the bodies' detoxification capacity. This has proven to be a major problem with vaccinations, where they are tested as a single shot, often in the doctors' offices they are given many at a time which is ever more dangerous.

In any detoxification or cleanse program, one must realize that the gastrointestinal track, liver and kidneys work to rid the body of toxins, thus a balanced detoxification program should be sought after.

An optimal cleanse program should be designed to:

- Stimulate and strengthen the GI tract with a focus to lessen toxin accumulation.

- Provide nutritional support which targets liver detoxification mechanisms and neutralizes toxins.

- Encourages and optimal acid-alkaline balance, providing regularity and enhancing toxin excretion.

There are a ton of cleanse and detoxification products on the market, but what you need to consider first is every day cleansing through food. That's right; food can actually act as a supporter of detoxification, from alkalinizing foods such as fruits and vegetables, to fiber, to cruciferous vegetables such as broccoli and Brussels sprouts providing the body the ability to convert estrogens to the preferable 2-hydroxy estrone metabolites we spoke of earlier.

When choosing a supplement for cleansing, especially if you are on medications, in addition to using quality supplements, it is important to clear the routine with your pharmacist or physician, since you might alter the metabolism of the medication which could alter blood levels.

"Chelation" is a popular term where it represents detoxifying heavy metals from the body. Where there are natural supplements that can support this in a gentle fashion, there are medications and treatments in physicians' offices which can detoxify heavy metals, or chelate them in a more aggressive manner. Only go through such a process with a qualified practitioner since chelation done in an improper manner can put a strain on the kidney's as well as leave the body deficient in minerals if not adequately replenished.

You will find many natural detoxification products on the market, here are a few ingredients I like to look for due to their natural detoxification properties for common, mild environmental exposures.

Modified Citrus Pectin- Shown to promote healthy urinary excretion of common environmental exposures such as mercury, arsenic, cadmium, lead and tin without altering excretion of other minerals, such as calcium, magnesium, iron, copper and selenium.

Cilantro and chlorella (as food or supplements) - Have a long history of traditional use in supporting the body's natural process for maintaining healthy metal levels.

N-acetyl-l-cysteine (NAC) – Shown to promote urinary excretion of methylmercury and provides support for the liver by enhancing glutathione (a potent antioxidant) concentration.

Milk thistle- Nutritionally supports liver function, supports glutathione concentrations and has antioxidant properties where it protects the liver from free radical damage.

L-glutamine- Helps to maintain healthy intestinal integrity, ensuring proper nutrient utilization while limiting the amount of toxins that pass through the intestinal barrier.

DIM (diindolymethane) and I3C (indole-3-carbinol) – Promote healthy estrogen metabolism.

Calcium-d-Glucarate- Shown to support the body's natural ability to detoxify internal and environmental toxins including estrogens.

Lastly, never detox if you are constipated, you will only recycle your toxins. Also, if you are on medications, understand that a detox can affect the levels of your medication in your system, thus blood pressure, other heart meds, diabetes meds, etc. could produce different results.

Checklist for Detoxification Support

1. Take steps to eliminate as much toxin exposure on a daily basis in relation to the sources mentioned above.
2. Diet. Avoid and limit as many dietary toxins including GMO's, pesticides, herbicide's, heavy metals, and even consider dairy and wheat. Incorporate natural detoxifying foods into ones diet.
3. Promote a healthy digestive tract with digestive enzymes and probiotics.
4. Never detoxify if constipated.

5. Supplements. Incorporating a combination of foundational nutrition as well as other supportive supplements can serve someone very well. I find supplements such as modified citrus pectin (Pectasol-C is one of my favorites.) Also, products with chlorella and cilantro such as Pures HM Chelate are also a good choice.

6. If problems still continue, or severe in nature, seek out a qualified practitioner in measures of assessing and treating toxic burdens.

See also: Digestive Health, Diet, Food Allergens and Intolerance's.

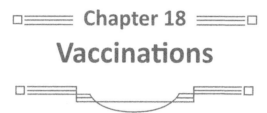

Chapter 18

Vaccinations

I was contemplating whether to address the topic of vaccinations in this book or not. It is such as enormous topic that complete books are written on the good, the bad and the ugly of vaccinations, and I will share with you some of my favorite resources including books, websites and other programs.

Due to the fact that more and more pharmacies and practitioners are promoting vaccination programs, I felt it would be a disservice to leave this topic out. I will look at the subject from a holistic point of view, because the problem is the way vaccine information is delivered via main-stream sources is not in a truth based, unbiased view.

So for this chapter, my goal is not to address each and every vaccine, or try to convince you if a certain vaccine is bad or good; but help you clear through the confusion and encourage you to do your due diligence to assess if vaccinations are appropriate for you and your family through known facts and relevant examples.

I have personally seen numerous cases of vaccine injury, whether to family members, friends and clients. Some have resulted in severe reactions affecting the child and family for a lifetime, others seemed to eradicate after a few days, months, or years, although where none the less highly concerning at the time. I have witnessed different reactions from the parents. Many have recognized the relationship and opted for limited or a ban on vaccinations for their children going forward, in other cases the response is one of disbelief, and almost a refusal to connect the dots. I think the latter is based on a subconscious reaction that a parent might feel responsible for, which is understandable.

Remember, this is all about self-responsibility, and transparency. On the other side of the coin I have seen people opting out of vaccinations for themselves and their children claiming they are unsafe and the cause of many diseases, while at the same time they take no responsibility for their own health and their own immunity- this is inexcusable in itself.

I think many would agree that an ultimate goal would be to have safe, effective and necessary vaccines, but sadly, this is often not the case. Personally I think the vaccination policies which have been created are nothing less than insane. Most vaccines are not based on good science; they are sold by fear through the media, the books are cooked on their necessity and effectiveness, and are even promoted through government based mandates.

The topic of vaccines causing autism often comes up. I have my personal feelings, and if you look at the biology of autism, than you will see why many consider it a an environmental disease of challenged detoxification. When I say environmental, I refer to the environment inside and outside the body. In other words, the body does not have the ability to detoxify chemicals and compounds which lead to brain and neurological damage. I am not making a claim here, although I often wonder with the push of adult vaccinations such as the shingles vaccine, Zostavax, if we will soon be seeing the escalation of Alzheimer's disease like we have Autism, considering all the toxic adjuvants which come in the vaccinations.

I don't find it a coincidence that as the amounts of vaccines that children receive have increased, so have the rates of autism, in fact, science backs this up. A study published in the *Journal of Toxicology and Environmental Health*, titled, *A positive association found between autism prevalence and childhood vaccination uptake across the U.S. population* affirms the relationship.

In this study, researchers recognize that individuals probably have a genetic predisposition to develop autism, although suspect that one or more environmental triggers are also needed. One of those triggers might be the battery of vaccinations that young children receive.

Through their research, a positive and statistically significant relationship was found: The higher the proportion of children receiving recommended vaccinations, the higher was the prevalence of autism or speech or language impairment. A 1% increase in vaccination was associated with an additional 680 children having autism or speech or language impairment. Neither parental behavior nor access to care affected the results, since vaccination proportions were not significantly related to any other disability or to the number of pediatricians in a U.S. state. The researchers concluded that the results suggest that although mercury has been removed from many vaccines, other culprits may link vaccines to autism.

Recent figures for autism prevalence amongst school-age children (2-17 years) in the United States were recently published in a report by the Centers for Disease Control (CDC). According to this new estimate, rates of autism amongst the nation's school children have climbed to 1 in 50, up from an estimated 1 in 88 for 2012, an increase partly represented by a broadening of the definition of autism, as well as increase in the ability to detect it.

You will see below that aside from mercury, which has garnished most of the attention as a toxin within a vaccine, there are many more toxins to challenge the body's immune system, and lead to overload. Did you know that the FDA safety level for aluminum exposure for an infant is 20 mcg (micrograms), and the Hepatitis B vaccine that is now given to newborns contains 225 mcg of aluminum? Aside from the fact that the Hepatitis B vaccine was originally created for IV drug users and people who were the sex profession due to high risk of contracting Hepatitis B and now are pawning them off on babies new to the world, aluminum is a neurotoxin and can lead to neurological injury.

Take a "simple" flu vaccine for example. Convince me where it is good science that a baby, or young child is recommended to receive the same amount and dose as an adult- yes, a baby or even pregnant mother would receive the same flu vaccine as Shaquille O'Neal. There is no good science to this and if this does not lead you to question the flu vaccine programs, I don't know what will.

I mentioned earlier how drug pipelines in many categories have been drying up, thus drug companies are looking towards integrative medicine and nutrition. Nutrition pales in comparison to the windfall of financial riches that the vaccination industry promises to drug companies involved. And where it shows financial promise, what I find ever so disgusting is the continued promotion in light of a multitude of vaccine side-effects and cases of vaccine injury arguably far outweighing any benefits.

We talked about the influence that drug companies over the entire healthcare system, including medical schools, medical journals, hospitals, clinics and the local pharmacy. Often times health care practitioners livelihoods depend on blind faith, without questioning any aspect of any vaccination. Many would argue this is what has created the industry of pediatricians, where aside from seeing patients on cases of cough and cold, much of their practices are based on "well care" visits which is essentially an appointment for vaccination boosters.

It seems even when obvious evidence of vaccine damage occurs right before a doctor's eyes, s/he is often unwilling to consider a vaccine as the cause. As I mentioned in a parents case of not wanting to face the fact that they might feel responsible, they turn that blind eye, could it not be the same for a physician?

More Vaccinations Proven To Be a Bad Thing

The recommended childhood vaccination schedule has increased dramatically over the years, and our children are no healthier for it. The Cal-Oregon vaccination survey which surveyed parents of 17,674 vaccinated vs. unvaccinated U.S. showed:

- Vaccinated children had 120% more asthma.

- Vaccinated boys had 317% more ADHD.

- Vaccinated boys had 185% more neurologic disorders.

- Vaccinated boys had 146% more autism.

The results of this study do not appear to be a fluke. An ongoing German survey released its own preliminary study back in September 2011. The study results show that children who have been vaccinated according to official government schedules are up to five times more likely to contract a preventable disease than children who developed their own immune systems naturally without vaccines.

The survey includes data on 8,000 unvaccinated children whose overall disease rates were compared to disease rates among the general population, the vast majority of which have been vaccinated. And in every single disease category, unvaccinated children fared far better than vaccinated children in terms of both disease prevalence and severity.

More Vaccinations at Once is Even Worse

If U.S. children receive all doses of all vaccines, they are injected with up to 35 shots that contain 113 different kinds of disease particles, 59 different chemicals, four types of animal cells/DNA, human DNA from aborted fetal tissue and human albumin. In many cases, doctors and nurses administer numerous vaccines all at once during a single visit to make sure children get all these shots and to save time.

According to data compiled from the government's *Vaccine Adverse Events Reporting System* (VAERS), as many as 145,000 children or more have died throughout the past 20 years as a result of this multiple vaccine dose approach, and few parents are aware of this shocking fact.

In a study published in the journal *Human & Experimental Toxicology*, researchers evaluated the overall number of hospitalizations and deaths associated with vaccines administered between 1990 and 2010, and compared this data to the number of vaccines given at one time to individual children. Upon analysis, the team found that the more vaccines a child receives during a single doctor visit, the more likely he or she is to suffer a severe reaction or even die. According to Heidi Stevenson from *Gaia Health*, for each additional vaccine a child receives his or her chance of death increases by an astounding 50 percent -- and with each additional vaccine dose, chances of having to be hospitalized for severe complications increase two-fold.

Oh, and one last think on childhood vaccinations. Remember in the beginning when I talked about the drug company GlaxoSmithKline pleading guilty to the largest drug industry scandal which resulted in 3 Billion dollars' worth of fines? It seems that as I am writing this, GSK has partnered with an India-based pharmaceutical company to develop a six-in-one, single dose vaccine. This is after a pentavalent (5-in-1) vaccine is being found responsible for numerous deaths through India in 2012 and 2013 alone. - This is absolutely unacceptable and health care providers can no longer be turning a blind eye to these facts. If you are presented with a multi-vaccine, one piece of information I feel comfortable in giving you is to run the other way.

Assessing The Need and Effectiveness of Vaccinations

Once again, I am not taking a stance of "no vaccinations," I believe it is your choice. What I want to do is give you what I feel is critical information to assess the needs for yourself.

When talking to people, I find that from commercials on television, people fall under the belief that there is a clear need to get certain vaccinations, and the vaccinations are 100% effective in preventing disease. This is a major problem, I believe deceitful, and a tool that is used to influence practitioners and the public on vaccines needs and effectiveness.

First off, did you know that a number of diseases were eradicated way before their vaccines were created?

Diptheria

The 1800's was a time when infectious disease was rampant, and what was needed was better measures of sanitation. Diptheria was quite a problem and to combat the number of people dying was what is called an antitoxin, which is designed to neutralize a specific toxin, such as diphtheria. This is different from a vaccination in that vaccines are purposed to prevent disease caused by toxins. One was created in the late 1800's and to give you an idea of its possible effectiveness, with the addition of what I believe increased sanitation, in 1900 there were approximately 40 deaths per 100,000 people from diphtheria.

By 1920 there were less than 20 deaths per 100,000 people, thus in a relative short time, the mortality rate was more than cut in half. 1920 was when the diphtheria vaccine was introduced, clearly after the "cleaning up" of the disease and eradication already begun.

Whooping Cough

Whooping cough hit its peak in mortality around 1918 with a rate of approximately 15 to 20 people dying per 100,000 each year. By the time the whooping cough vaccine was introduced in the late 1940's, deaths from whooping cough were almost non-existent. In many cases, the recent whooping cough outbreaks over the last few years were predominately in those children who received the vaccine, not the unvaccinated. Where we cannot say that the whooping cough vaccine was the cause of the disease, one might suggest that with research backing that those who get more vaccinations get more illnesses, thus a compromised immune system which the vaccine could have further influenced.

Measles

There are countless examples to this day how natural immunity works wonderful for cases of the measles. You might even hear about "measles parties" where parents bring together their children who have not yet had the measles and are unvaccinated to acquire a natural immunity. Time and time again, reports show this to be a safe and effective alternative.

The heyday for measles deaths was around 1918 with about 15 deaths per 100,000 people. The measles vaccine was not introduced until 1963 when deaths from measles was once again, not an issue, problem already eradicated.

Cooking The Books- How To Influence Your Beliefs Through Numbers

Giving the fact that vaccines are not free of side-effects, this to me is totally unconscionable and gives both the business of marketing as well as the morals of our medical system a black eye.

Here is an example of a vaccine that has gained great popularity over recent years. Zostavax is a vaccine that is promoted to prevent shingles in adults. If you go to the Zostavax website or watch a commercial, chances are that you will walk away with the feeling that shingles are very common, if you get shingles you will get the debilitating neurological pains, and that the vaccine is 100% able to prevent you from getting shingles. When I began writing this chapter, the Zostavax website promoted the fact that the vaccine has an efficacy rate of 70%, which would make one think that if you lined 100 people up, gave them all the vaccine, that it would prevent shingles in 70 of them. Incidentally, I see they changed their website around and are not making such as blatant claim, let me show you why I think this is so.

The website alluded to a study titled, Efficacy, Safety, and Tolerability of Herpes Zoster Vaccine in Persons Aged 50-59 Years.

Here is how they got their numbers. This study enrolled 22,439 individuals between the ages of 50-59 years of age. 11,211 received the vaccination, while 11,228 received a placebo. And keep in mind, the 50-59 age group is not a common age group to get shingles, thus the chances of acquiring the disease are low to begin with, which as you will see, influences their numbers.

Of the 11,211 who received the vaccination, 30 people got shingles.

Of the 11,228 who received the placebo, 99 people got singles.

I called the company to ask how they came about a 70% efficacy rate with these numbers and they told me, "subtracting the 30 people who acquired shingles and received the vaccine from the 99 people who got shingles and did not receive the vaccine, leaves a difference of 69, thus "approximately a 70% efficacy rate."

Do you see how these numbers are misrepresenting the facts?

First, if you take the 11,228 who received the placebo and divide by those who contracted shingles, this gives only a .8% rate of acquiring shingles of those 50 to 59 years old, hardly something to be worried about.

And I agree, studying the 50 to 59 year olds is not an appropriate age group to study, as singles becomes more common as one gets older, certainly above the 60 year old range, where some estimates are 50% of those over 80 years old can acquire shingles.

So, let's take a look at the broad average. The CDC believes that 1 out of 3 people will acquire herpes zoster (shingles) in their lifetime, and the risk of developing the emotionally triggering and painful post-herpetic neuralgia (PHN), is 10% to 18%.

So, if you line up 100 adults, and 1/3 develop herpes zoster, which would be approximately 33 people, and let's take an average of 15% developing post-herpetic neuralgia as an average, then out of every 100 people, 4.95, so let's say 5 will develop the painful shingles.

Heck, if the vaccine is 100% effective, all well and good you might say, but the numbers certainly do not back this up.

So let's take a look at effectiveness from the point of view of how many vaccinations need to be given to prevent 1 case of shingles, or "The Number Needed to Treat (NNT)." For this I would like to look at another study, titled, A Vaccine To Prevent Herpes Zoster and Postherpetic Neuralgia in Older Adults, published in the New England Journal of Medicine, June 2005.

I like this study because it is larger and focuses in on the age group of 60 and older, for whom developing shingles is of greater incidence.

This was a study of 38,546 individuals over the age of 60, and over 95% of them completed the study, thus we will use 36,618 for our numbers (95% of 38,546.) This study went on for a little over 3 years.

Of the 36,618 individuals who finished the study, 957 came down with shingles, 315 from the vaccinated group, and 642 from the placebo. Then by subtracting 315 from 642 which equals 327, gives us the number of cases prevented. From this we will divide 36, 618 by 327 to give us our number needed to treat (NNT), which is 111. So in this study you need to vaccinate 111 people to prevent one case of shingles- hardly a set of numbers that makes me feel comfortable.

And as you know, in medicine, the financial expense is a major issue. So taking into account each shingles vaccine costs $200 (a cost to either the individual, insurance company, or government program), it costs $22,200 to prevent one case of shingles.

Given the numbers, I don't know if I am convinced for the mass vaccination approach that our medical system takes. To show you that this "number influencing" is not an isolated case, let's take a look at the flu vaccine.

The Flu Vaccine

In my mind the flu vaccination program is nothing more than a manipulative marketing campaign sold off of fear. I constantly have patients ask me if I believe in getting the flu vaccine. My answer is, "it's not for me; I rather support my immune system, but do your own research and make your own choice."

Where the flu vaccine might not seem to be the most dangerous of vaccinations, I question the necessity, as well as the science. As you probably know, it's based off a guess of what strains will be active in the upcoming season, it's full of 'inactive' ingredients posing possible harm, and as I write this at the end of the 2012-2013 flu season which the CDC has called the worst flu pandemic in a decade, I have seen many customers acquire the flu despite receiving the flu shot. All the while you continually hear doctor's offices and pharmacies promoting the flu shot. And yes, my guess is that many believe that it works (in addition to it being a profit center), but to not be educated or offered an alternative in naturally supporting your immune system- that is unconscionable.

Let's take a look at how numbers are manipulated as we did with the shingles vaccine above. Back in the fall of 2011, the CDC reported on a study published in the medical journal, The Lancet, saying that the flu vaccine has a 60% effectiveness rate. The study was titled, Efficacy and effectiveness of influenza vaccines: a systematic review and meta-analysis. Hearing "60% effectiveness rate", one would think that for every 100 people vaccinated, 60 would have the flu prevented, right? Here's the thing, when you look at the study, it actually reveals that the flu vaccine only prevents influenza in 1.5 out of 100 adults injected, thus the 60% seems a bit sketchy. Let's see how the numbers unfold this time.

The basis of the real numbers comes from metrics in the review itself, that only about 2.7 in 100 adults get the first place. So, once again, the relevant population is misinterpreted as we saw in the shingles vaccine.

This being a meta-analysis, means researchers studied the results of multiple different studies which already took place on efficacy of the flu vaccine.

In the analysis there were 13,095 adults who did not receive the vaccine. Of these 13,095 individuals, 347 of them came down with influenza. By dividing 347 by 13,095, this means that only 2.7% of not vaccinated even caught the flu. This alone leaves me to question the need for a mass vaccination program, do you agree?

Of those who received the vaccine, 1.2% did not catch the flu.

So, now let's look to see how they came up with a 60% effectiveness rate when it is obvious that the chances of catching the flu are quite low, regardless.

What do we know now?

2.7% of those who did not have the flu shot, got the flu.

1.2% of those who got the flu shot got the flu.

The difference between these two groups is 1.5%, pointing to the fact that out of every 100 people vaccinated, only 1.5 are prevented from getting the flu. Thus in this example, the Number Needed to Vaccinate to prevent one case of the flu is approximately 66 people. (By dividing 100 by 1.5 you get 66.6)

Gardasil and Cervarix

One of the biggest markets of recent years in regards to vaccinations is HPV (human papilloma virus) vaccines. There has been many a collusion between drug companies and local, state and even Federal agencies in the U.S. and abroad in regards to mandates, forcing females, sometimes even males, to receive the vaccine, at times even without the consent of their parents. You cannot tell me this is good medicine.

Side-effects of the HPV Vaccines are many, including deaths and being permanently disabled as you will see below. But before we even get into the side-effect profiles, let's see how relevant an HPV vaccine really is, and examine if it is even effective.

The HPV vaccine is sold like many other vaccines under emotions and tactics of fear. The assertion or marketing line that you are told is that the HPV vaccine prevents cervical cancer. First off, cervical cancer is one of the rarest forms of cancer, and there is no evidence that HPV alone can cause cervical cancer, it would have to be as a co-infection with one or more of the many different risk factors to cervical such as cytomegalovirus, Epstein Barr virus, chlamydia and others.

Over the past forty years, regular pap smear testing has shown to prevent cervical cancer by over 74%, thus if a female got regular pap smears the chances of getting cervical cancer are less than 2000'ths of one percent.

Not to minimalize those affected by cervical cancer, but did you know that there are only 12,000 cases of cervical cancers per year, and 4,000 deaths?

Having HPV does not mean getting cancer. There are over 100 strains of HPV, 15 are known to cause cancer, and the HPV vaccines only target two of these strains. And, when detected, HPV infection is easily managed and rarely proceeds to cancer regardless of the strain.

Now what if I was to tell you that the HPV vaccines have never been proven to prevent cervical cancer, and that the vaccine was fast tracked for FDA approval, avoiding many of the astringent testing on safety and efficacy that other drugs and vaccines endure? After taking a look at the reported side-effects I think you will find it obvious not to automatically sign off on your son or daughter getting the vaccine.

Below are the statistics of adverse reactions related to the HPV Vaccine from VAERS Reports as of January, 2013. In addition to the alarming rates of side effects and cases of vaccine injury including death and permanent disablement, keep in mind that research shows that only 2 to 10% of any adverse reactions actually gets reported, the vast majority are not. Taking this into account, and realizing the low numbers of cervical cancer cases, deaths related to cervical cancers and questionable efficacy, it is apparent that benefits do not outweigh the risks.

To put the *"nail in the coffin"* on this debate, I would like to share with you words from the lead researcher, Dr. Diane Harper, on the safety and effectiveness of Gardasil.

Dr. Diane Harper helped design and carry out the Phase II and Phase III safety and effectiveness studies to get Gardasil approved, and authored many of the published, scholarly papers about it. She has been a paid speaker and consultant to Merck.

At the 4th International Public Conference on Vaccination, which took place in Reston, Virginia on Oct. 2nd through 4th, 2009, Dr. Harpers speech was supposed to promote the Gardasil and Cervarix vaccines, but she threw everyone a curveball and basically spoke out against the vaccines.

Dr. Harper explained in her presentation that the cervical cancer risk in the U.S. is already extremely low, and that vaccinations are unlikely to have any effect upon the rate of cervical cancer in the United States. In fact, 70% of all H.P.V. infections resolve themselves without treatment in a year, and the number rises to well over 90% in two years. Dr. Harper also mentioned the safety angle. All trials of the vaccines were done on children aged

15 and above, despite them currently being marketed for 9-year-olds. Dr. Harper claimed that she was speaking out, so that she might finally be able to sleep at night.

What about prevention? It is well known that lifestyle risk factors such as diet can dramatically increase ones chances of developing cervical cancers. Aside from measures of healthy diet and life style, nutrition has been shown to play a role. Supplements such as vitamin c, curcumin, quercetin and other bioflavonoids have shown to contribute to reductions of HPV infections and cervical cancer. In fact, studies done in underdeveloped countries such as India have shown those who consume the highest intake of B12 and Folic Acid have a 79% reduction in HPV infections and cervical cancer than those with low intake.

Description	Total
Disabled	924
Deaths	130
Did Not Recover	5,736
Abnormal Pap Smear	515
Cervical Dysplasia	203
Cervical Cancer	61
Life Threatening	543
Emergency Room	10,225
Hospitalized	2,911
Extended Hospital Stay	229
Serious	3,901
Adverse Events	28,661

This is another perfect example of how prevention is worth way more than a pound of cure.

Harmful Inactive Ingredients

One of the main concerns over vaccines is the questionably harmful 'inactive' ingredients. This has urged a movement and demand for what are known as 'green vaccines.' Why don't these pharmaceutical companies create green vaccines, free of known dangerous excipients? It will raise costs, decrease profits, and most likely lead to an increase in out of pocket expenses to the patient, possibly resulting in patients less willing to roll up their sleeves so easily.

But let's just take a look at some of the ingredients in conventional vaccines, and I ask you, how can these not be harmful?

- Stray viruses and bacteria from the animal cell cultures that vaccines are made in.
- Mercury, a well-documented neurotoxin, is still in the multi-dose flu vaccines throughout the world. Trace amounts remain in several other vaccines.
- Aluminum, a poison that can cause bone, bone marrow and brain degeneration.
- Animal cells from monkeys, dog kidneys, chickens, cows, and humans.
- Formaldehyde (embalming fluid), a known carcinogen.
- Polysorbate 80, known to cause infertility in female mice and testicular atrophy in male mice.
- Gelatin, from pigs and cows, known to cause anaphylactic reactions, is found in large quantities in the MMR, chickenpox and shingles vaccines.
- Monosodium glutamate (MSG), an excitotoxin in inhaled flu vaccines, is known to cause metabolic disturbances (e.g. diabetes), seizures and other neurologic disorders. Think about it, you are placing MSG inches from the brain.

Side-effects and examples of vaccine injury documented in medical literature and/or in package inserts:

- Arthritis
- Bleeding disorders, blood clots, sepsis
- Heart attacks
- Ear infections
- Fainting (with reports of broken bones)
- Miscarriages
- Narcolepsy
- Kidney failure requiring dialysis
- Seizures/epilepsy
- Severe allergic reactions, such as hives and anaphylaxis
- Sudden death
- Neurological disorders

Disease states that have documented associations with vaccines:

- Allergies and eczema
- Arthritis
- Asthma
- Autism
- Acid reflux requiring an infant to take proton pump inhibitors, which have many side effects
- Cancer
- Diabetes (infant and childhood)
- Kidney disease
- Neurological disease
- Autoimmune diseases
- Sudden Infant Death Syndrome (SIDS)

Due to these adverse reactions, side-effects, disease states and examples of vaccine injury, there is a fund created, where a portion of every vaccine sale goes into what is known as the National Vaccine Injury Compensation Program (NVICP). The NVICP has awarded more than $1.2 billion in damages to children and adults injured by vaccines, nearly $ 6 million to victims of the HPV vaccines. So if you can say to yourself that this does not require more evaluations based on safety, that the medical community and drug industry at large has our nation's health in mind, you might be fooling yourself.

And there is so much further we can go, but what has happened is that the line between what is credible and what is fear based manipulative information has become so blurred that many people are left in a state of confusion and often overwhelmed on what decisions to make for the good of themselves and their families.

One response I often hear is that "they won't let my child into school without vaccination" and this is not a fact. Understand that exemptions do exist in almost every state, whether be based on religious views, health, or personal beliefs- vaccinations are not mandatory. Although as I mentioned, every state has different rules and what applies, so it is important to do some homework to find what applies where you live.

To further clear the confusion about vaccination here are some resources:

Web resources for more information and help

- **Mary Tocco**
  www.childhoodshots.com
- **Dr. Sherri Tenpenny**
  www.drtenpenny.com
- **SaneVax** - *www.sanevax.org*
- **Global Vaccine Institute**
  www.thinktwice.com
- **Dr. Rashi Buttar**
  http://www.drbuttar.com/

Books for more information and a place to start

- Global Vaccine Institute
  www.thinktwice.com

- *DVD or CD- Are Vaccines Safe? - Mary Tocco*

- *Saying No To Vaccines* – Sherri Tenpenny, DO

- *Make an Informed Vaccine Decision For the Health of Your Child* – Mayer Eisenstein, MD, JD, MPH

- *Vaccines: Are They Really Safe and Effective?* – Neil Miller

- *Childhood Vaccinations: Questions All Parents Should Ask* – Tedd Koren, DC

- *How to Raise a Healthy Child in Spite of Your Doctor* – Robert Mendelsohn, MD

- *Natural Alternatives to Vaccination* – Zoltan Rona, MD

- *The Sanctity of Human Blood: Vaccination is Not Immunization* – Tim O'Shea, DC

And to finish up this chapter, I would like to answer a question I have not yet heard an answer to, and often stumps the folks that I ask, especially when fingers are pointed at the unvaccinated:

"If vaccinations worked so well, why would the unvaccinated be a threat to vaccinated?"

Chapter 19

The Crimes We Commit Against Our Stomachs

The digestive tract is one of the most important systems of your body, and in our culture, often one of the most abused. The digestive tract plays a role in all areas of health and wellness, and is critical to dial in other disease states with healthy digestive and enzymatic activity to ensure that nutrients are being digested and assimilated, and toxins are released.

Prescription and over the counter medications for digestive disorders account for one of the most common classes of drugs prescribed, and you guessed it, they can come with some major challenges against one's health. Issues such as gastric reflux, heart burn, constipation, diarrhea and gas are merely symptoms, and when we are treating only the symptoms we are opening the body up to a host of other problems including irritable bowel syndrome (IBS), dysbiosis, candida, autoimmune disease states such as Ulcerative Colitis and Crohn's Disease and even colorectal cancer, the second most common form of cancer.

The digestive tract has many roles including: digestion of foods, break down nutrients for energy, critical relationship with one's immune system, detoxification, hormone metabolism, manufacturers' vitamins and mood elevating neurotransmitter's, natural antibiotics and more. So as you can see, if the digestive tract becomes impaired or falls victim to a disease state, the effects can be noticed throughout the body.

Let's take a look at one of the most common digestive complaints, which can often snowball into many of the other disease states above if treated incorrectly or not at all, which is acid reflux and heart-burn.

Acid Reflux and Heart-burn

In Conventional Medicine the answer to treating acid reflux has been to neutralize, reduce or block our natural hydrochloric acid (HCL) production and release in the body. One must keep in mind, a symptom such as acid reflux could be a sign of a greater problem brewing, and thus quieting the symptom might not be the best option. As you will see, there is a reason that most of the over the counter packages for acid reflux such as Prilosec® and Prevacid® come with a warning that they are only indicated for short term use.

Even though these medications are not approved for long term use, doctors will prescribe for the long term, most pharmacists will dispense with out the warnings of long term therapy, and being that many of these drugs are purchased without prescriptions, and patients take them indefinitely, often not knowing the problems that they can cause.

If you have ever experienced acid reflux or heartburn, then you know it is one of the most uncomfortable feelings- and you will do almost anything to make it go away.

Not only is it uncomfortable, it can actually cause some damage to the esophageal lining if left alone too long, which might open up a short term treatment of some anti-acid medications. One must be aware though at the same time, the drugs (prescription and non-prescription) used to treat acid reflux can lead to, or influence issues such as escalated digestive disorders, impaired immunity and osteoporosis.

What many people do not realize is that a large portion of folks who suffer from heartburn and acid reflux do so due to too little hydrochloric acid (HCL) secretion, and not too much. HCL production and secretion can be suppressed due to lifestyle, diet, and stress. This is why the old wives tale of taking apple cider vinegar often helps to relive reflux since we are adding an acid to the system.

But, before you go downing apple cider vinegar, let's take a closer look into what might be going on, and how to better support it.

The body uses the HCL it produces for a number of purposes. HCL acts as a primary defense against food borne pathogens and helps promote a healthy microbial balance. (Good bacteria (probiotics) –vs. - yeasts, bad bacteria, and even parasites). HCL helps the body digest, absorb and assimilate proteins, calcium, vitamin B12, and iron.

Acid reducing medications can deplete nutrients from your system including calcium, magnesium, B vitamins, vitamin D, iron, zinc, and more, you can see how long term treatment of this symptom could be adding insult to injury.

Thus as you can see, by the drug induced nutrient depletions as well as by reducing or altering the gastric pH over the long term, can lead to increasing digestive infections, impaired immunity, decreased nutritional status and influence issues of osteopenia and osteoporosis.

In fact, a recent study was just released showing that proton pump inhibitor's (Prilosec, Nexium, Prevacid, Protonix and others) increases the chance of Clostridum Difficile Diarrhea (Often referred to as C diff or CDAD) by 65%, and that's only taken for a few months.

What are the alternatives?

First of all, do not stop taking an acid reducing or neutralizing drug if it was recommended by your doctor. I mentioned previously that for the most part they are only indicated for the short term use, although there reasons they can be prescribed for the long term under a doctor's supervision. Thus in such instances, balancing the drug induced nutrient depletions such as calcium, magnesium, B vitamins and vitamin D might be the best option.

Although, if you are self-medicating, or would like to speak to your physician about alternative options, here is what I might recommend:

Reason would suggest supplementing with HCL, which is often a great option, although due to issues such as known or unknown digestive ulcers or even people taking medications such as anti-inflammatories and steroids, I like to consider a more conservative approach first.

There are a number of natural options for reflux and heartburn, as well as advanced therapies which we could look at for getting rid of bad organisms such as bacteria, viruses, yeast and parasites which don't belong. For this conversation I would like to stick with the foundational elements of (1) supporting the digestive process, (2) recolonize good bacteria (3) sooth and promote the integrity of the digestive lining, which can all help support common digestive symptoms of gas, indigestion, acid reflux, heartburn, diarrhea and constipation.

In stimulating and supporting the digestive process we are looking at supplements such as digestive enzymes, including amylase, which helps digest sugars, protease to digest proteins, and lipase to help digests fats.

Recolonizing good bacteria through probiotics is imperative, even in a healthy digestive tract where symptoms are not prevalent. We recommend high quality probiotics which have been tested to ensure that they will stick to the intestinal linings and actually colonize in the digestive tract. We support multi strain products as well, offering an array of acidophilus and bifidus strains to ensure colonization in both the large and small intestines.

To repair, sooth, and support the integrity there are a number of great natural ingredients including DGL (deglycyrrhizinated licorice), aloe, slippery elm, marshmallow root, glutamine, Sea cure®, and zinc carnosine, to name a few. These can be found alone or in combination supplements.

GMO's and The Gut

We already spoke of the devastation that GMO's (genetically modified organisms) can have on our health and environment, and it all starts in the gut. We spoke about how they disrupt the shikamate pathway which is present in the bacteria in our digestive tracts. Refer back to Chapter 7, for more on this topic, although if you are dealing with any digestive disorders, it is imperative to navigate towards a GMO free diet.

Cancer Therapy and the Gut

One area that there could be a huge benefit in implementing complementary therapy is in the area of cancer therapy. There are both natural and conventional treatments of cancer, and where this conversation is not about which is better, safer, etc., I would like to talk about the challenges of chemotherapy and radiation on the gastrointestinal tract.

Both chemotherapy and radiation can damage the health of the digestive tract; inclusive of destroying good bacteria which should exist in the digestive tract and is a major part of a healthy immune system, as well as damaging the epithelial lining of the intestines leading to micro-tares which could be responsible for the leaking of toxins into the blood stream as well as challenging optimal nutrient absorption.

For people who have undergone or are undergoing chemotherapy and/or ration, supplementation of L-Glutamine to support the integrity of the intestines, as well as probiotics to help recolonize good bacteria could serve an incredible benefit.

The Gut and Autism and Beyond

In the last chapter on vaccinations where we talked about autism, I referred to it as a disease of impaired detoxification. Time and time again, in integrative treatments to support the health of someone with autism, one of the primary actions taken is to heal the gut. One major take home, the quicker you act- the better.

Healing the gut has a storied past in the debate of the relationship between vaccinations and autism, and thanks to the work and steadfastness of Dr. Andrew Wakefield, we now know that a healthy digestive tract plays an enormous role in bringing a patient with autism (and frankly any disease) back to better health.

Dr. Andrew Wakefield is a British physician whom the fear based medical system has attempted to use as a target to discredit an openly balanced approach to health.

The short of the story is that while practicing in the United Kingdom, Dr. Wakefield began to notice a link between patients with autism and a very unhealthy and inflamed gastrointestinal tract. This led him to create his own small study in 1998 on the matter and he concluded a relationship with the MMR (measles, mumps and rubella) vaccine. This eventually led to his exile as a practicing physician in the United Kingdom to the United States.

Fast forward to 2011, the research done by Dr. Wakefield in his 1998 study was targeted and called faulty and manipulated, blaming him on trying to make some money on a gastrointestinal test he is involved in. Journalists at the British Medical Journal led the attack, and I think Dr. Wakefields response speaks volumes of the situation:

> "The British Medical Journal and reporter Brian Deer recently alleged that my 1998 research paper was 'a hoax' and 'an elaborate fraud' and that my motivation was profit.

> "I want to make one thing crystal clear for the record - my research and the serious medical problems found in those children were not a hoax and there was no fraud whatsoever. Nor did I seek to profit from our findings.

"I stand by the Lancet paper's methodology and the results which call for more research into whether environmental triggers cause gastrointestinal disease and developmental regression in children. In fact, despite media reports to the contrary, the results of my research have been duplicated in five other countries.

"It is not unexpected to see poor reporting and misinformation coming from Brian Deer, the lead reporter of the recent BMJ coverage. But to see coverage in other media that cites Deer's shoddy journalism in the BMJ as a final justification to claim there is no link between vaccines and autism is ludicrous. The MMR is only one vaccine of the eleven vaccinations on the pediatric schedule that has been studied for causing developmental problems such as autism. That is fact, not opinion. Any medical professional, government official or journalist who states that the case is closed on whether vaccines cause autism is jumping to conclusions without the research to back it up.

"I continue to fully support more independent research to determine if environmental triggers, including vaccines, are causing autism and other developmental problems. The current rate of autism is 1 in 110 children in the United States and 1 in 64 children in the U.K. My goal has always been and will remain the health and safety of children. Since the Lancet paper, I have lost my job, my career and my country. To claim that my motivation was profit is patently untrue. I will not be deterred - this issue is far too important."

As Dr. Wakefield mentioned, numerous studies have pointed to a link between the MMR vaccine and autism and bowel disease in children. For instance, in 2011, a study out of Wake Forest University School of Medicine examined 275 children with regressive autism and bowel disease- and at one point, of the 82 tested, 70 prove positive for the measles virus. And according to the team's leader, Dr. Stephen Walker, "Of the handful of results we have in so far, all are vaccine strain and none are wild measles."

In regards to Dr. Wakefields and others studies, this further supports that in the gastrointestinal tract of a number of children who have been diagnosed with regressive autism, there is evidence of a vaccine induced measles virus.

What I find interesting is this came on top of other unrelated research early the same week, indicating that children who have one course of antibiotics before the age of four, are almost twice as likely to develop IBS (irritable bowel syndrome) and three and one half times more at risk to develop crohns disease.

What this shows is that we as a culture are pummeling children with challenges to their health, and we really need to wake up and speak up to protect them, and the digestive track is ground zero.

And this does not just have its place in autism, the digestive tract has far reaching influence over the whole body and supporting the digestive process and healing the gut applies to numerous disease states including digestive disorders such as leaky gut, fibromyalgia, immune health, and more.

What do I mean by 'healing the gut?'

There can be a number of different ways to go about it, although what I would like to share with you is a protocol from a pharmaceutical grade nutraceutical company, Metagenics. They have outlined what they call The Four R's of Digestive Health…and regardless of what natural ingredients or nutritional company you may use, I feel their description offers an excellent explanation on how to "heel" the gut.

Remove

Remove refers to the removal of any gastrointestinal parasites and/or undesirable pathogens (bacteria or fungi) that may be present and contributing to dysfunction and/or abnormal symptoms. Remove also refers to the removal from the diet of allergens and intolerant foods and substances.

Replace

Replace denotes the replacement of any digestive factors (enzymes, for example) the body may not be making, or which it may be making in inadequate amounts. HCL (hydrochloric acid) which we spoke about previously, is a supplement you should take with meals. Most of us produce less of this as we get older. Pathogens such as Candida Albicans tend to flourish when HCL production is low. Digestive Enzymes are also very helpful especially when eating cooked foods.

Reinoculate

Reinoculate refers to the reintroduction of "friendly" or desirable gastrointestinal bacteria through the use of probiotics as we spoke of above.

Repair

Repair refers to nutrients which need to be provided for cellular repair and functioning of the gastrointestinal mucosal cells. In a normal, healthy intestine, the friendly bacteria produce molecules which directly nourish the cells lining the intestinal wall. With the loss of the beneficial bacteria, the cells lining the intestine literally starve to death and small gaps between cells are created. This allows the transport of toxins such as undigested food particles and pathogens into the blood stream. This is known as leaky gut and can lead to allergies, fatigue, IBS, and other chronic conditions.

Checklist for Digestive Support

1. **Diet.** Often modern-day diets are lacking in essential digestive enzymes due to being highly processed or consisting of foods which are primarily cooked. Consider incorporating more live foods such as fresh vegetables in one's diet which come with natural enzymes. Additionally, many people might be lacking in hydrochloric acid from issues such as diets predominate in cooked foods, as well as stress. One might consider supplementation with digestive enzymes, and/or hydrochloric acid (do not use in cases of digestive ulcers.)

2. **Avoid GMO's.** Due to the challenges GMO's present to digestive tracts, it is recommended to eat organic, and avoid GMO's.

3. **Incorporate quality probiotic supplementation on a regular basis.** Some of our favorites are Probiotic G.I. from Pure Encapsulations, or Dr. Ohhira's Professional blend.

4. If still experiencing problems, considering seeing a qualified practitioner to adequately incorporate the 4 R's mentioned above.

See also: Stress, Detoxification, Diet.

Chapter 20

Living Lobotomies – The Over Prescribing of Anti-Depressants and ADHD Medications

The prescribing of families of antipsychotics, anti-depressants, ADD and ADHD drugs have skyrocketed over the last 30 years. This is one area I wish more and more people would look more towards the help of someone who helps them talk things out, such as a psychologist, and not just resort to the prescribing of medication. I think when someone is given the ability to prescribe a prescription they often overlook some basic but very effective therapies such as the power of working through things, and not avoiding. The pen is not an almighty sword; I feel it is often an all-mighty short-cut.

In my own clinical nutrition practice I was there to assess and balance someone nutritionally and hormonally, although I often found what people were looking for was to be heard. This is a major problem in our medical system, people are not heard, and I don't say this is the fault of the practitioners. Where our medical system is designed around how low an insurance carrier can pay a practitioner, the practitioner does not have the time to spend with the patient.

The power to talk to someone who can help someone deal with what's really going on, address the subconscious and conscious root causes instead of covering them over with potent medications is a very powerful thing. All too often prescribers of all modalities, general practitioners, pediatricians, internists and psychiatrists go right to prescribing of very powerful, brain bending medications as if they are simple sugar pills.

Now, I understand there are many people with some very deep psychological wounds that might need the careful help with medication therapy, although for your average person feeling blue, I don't think this is often the course to follow- especially what's being done to children who do not have the voice to speak up for themselves. And regardless of one's degree of depression, providing someone with foundational elements of care such as psychological and nutritional and hormonal support in addition to or in lieu of medication therapy can offer an incredible benefit.

When mentioning foundational nutrition, we must not overlook vitamin D. Vitamin D is made in our skin from the interaction of cholesterol and sunshine. Our medical system tells us to lower our cholesterol and stay out of the sun. Therefore, it makes perfect sense that many of us are deficient in vitamin D, which has long been known to improve mood, a core issue with Seasonal Affective Disorder?

In fact, a recent study was released where they found low vitamin D levels in chronically depressed people. The most recent study entitled "The association between low vitamin D and depressive disorders," was published in the journal *Molecular Psychiatry*. The researchers used participants from the *Netherlands Study of Depression and Anxiety* (NESDA).

They used the standard 25(OH) D serum level measurements and one-third of this group had low serum vitamin D readings by their standard, which is actually slightly different than those in the United States. The European Union uses 50 nmol/L (nanomols per liter), which translates to 20 ng/ml (nanograms per milliliter). American endocrinologists consider less than 30 ng/ml deficient.

More progressive medical practitioners claim blood serum readings should be 40 ng/ml – 60 ng/ml.

Medications That Know No Boundaries

I mentioned children, and this is of grave concern, and a very big problem we see every day. Prescribing medications which were once meant for adults are now being prescribed to children. This "off label" use of very powerful prescription drugs can come with a host of dangerous side effects-effects equal to or worse than the behavioral problems they are supposedly treating.

In a study published in the *Archives of General Psychiatry*, data from the National Ambulatory Medical Care Surveys from 1993 to 2009, found that doctor visits between 1993-1998 and 2005-2009 that involved a prescription of antipsychotic medication for children jumped sevenfold.

Furthermore, while children and adolescents show higher rates of antipsychotic prescription increases than adults, overall every age bracket is being prescribed more antipsychotics today than in previous years. Many of the prescriptions written to these children weren't even written by psychiatrists, but general practitioners who haven't been trained specifically in behavioral, cognitive, or mental disorders.

One of the head researchers to this study suggested that more needs to be done to increase access and availability of psychosocial interventions. "Parent management training and cognitive problem-solving skills training are examples of effective but underused treatments for young people with disruptive behavioral problems," he said.

What your doctors and pharmacists will often not tell you is that in controlling behavior, antipsychotics act on the frontal lobes of the brain -- the same area of the brain targeted by a lobotomy.

Dr. Peter Breggin, a psychiatrist from Ithaca, N.Y., an outspoken critic of widespread antipsychotic use in children, said these drugs damage developing brains.

"This is a situation where we have ruined the brains of millions of children." "These are lobotomizing drugs," he added. "Of course, they will reduce all behavior, including irritability," he said.

Recent data suggests that 1 in 10 Americans are on some sort of antidepressant medication. The Center for Disease Control and Prevention (CDC) released a report in 2011 that showed a dramatic increase in the use of antidepressants in Americans from 2005 to 2008. The CDC report claims that 11% of Americans over the age of 12 take antidepressant medications.

In addition, women are far more likely to take antidepressant medication than men at all levels of depression severity. The CDC data also revealed that 23% of women in their 40's and 50's take an SSRI. This is higher than any other age group and not surprising as we have mentioned that we are becoming hormonally exhausted and imbalanced such as with progesterone at earlier ages. I have seen numerous times when someone's hormonal imbalances are addressed; chemical antidepressants are no longer needed.

The symptoms of depression can include sadness, fatigue, irritability, apathy, feelings of isolation, loss of interest in favorite activities, hopelessness, insomnia, significant weight changes, aches and pains, and even thoughts of death and suicide. Look back on the chapter on hormones; from adrenal health to progesterone, estrogen and testosterone, we talked about many of the symptoms of hormonal balance which could lead to many of these symptoms.

Nutritional deficiencies can also be the cause of depression, thus opening up the ability of natural supplements to provide support for this disorder. Nutritional deficiencies linked with depression include the B vitamins, particularly, B1 (thiamine), B2 (riboflavin), B6 (pyridoxine), B7 (biotin), B9 (folic acid), and B12 (cobalamin), calcium, copper, iron, magnesium, vanadium, zinc and fatty acids.

Looking back on the chapter on drug induced nutrient depletions, where this was just a small sample of nutrients depleted by commonly prescribed medications, you can see how b vitamins are depleted through birth control pills and oral estrogens, B 12 by metformin, magnesium by blood pressure medications, and calcium by medications used for heart-burn; thus can you see how looking a bit more holistically can have an impact on someone's wellbeing?

One's diet can play a dramatic role in mood support. We have talked about the benefits of having an alkalinizing diet and one of those benefits is a positive mood. An acidic pH can leave someone moody, short tempered, feeling blue; thus the importance of a diet which is alkaline forming, abundant in vegetables and fruits, and even supplementation to ensure an adequate mineral status. One should also realize that medications are generally acidifying to ones pH, add to this the fact that many will deplete pH alkalinizing minerals is like adding insult to injury.

In the area of general antidepressants form common drugs such as the selective serotonin reuptake inhibitors (SSRI's) such as Prozac, Paxil, Zoloft and others, I have seen people go on a merry-go-round of drug therapy, after a year one drug does not work, they switch to another one which might stimulate slightly different receptors. The result is that drugs alone are not the answer.

Because depression can not only have a great impact on daily life, and even lead to suicide, it is important to consult a physician who can adequately assess the whole body, including issues of nutritional deficiencies.

ADD/ADHD

In the chapter on food intolerances and food allergies, we talked about how food intolerances, food additives and food colorings can lead to a child acting out, experiencing hyper-excitability and symptoms which can lead to a diagnosis of ADD and ADHD. Other factors which can lead to issues of ADD and ADHD include brain injury, toxin exposure, metal toxicities, pre-natal fatty acid deficiencies, and nutritional deficiencies.

Another major issue I see with children being put on these powerful medicines is that it seems that the system is not built for them. They are often highly intelligent, and/or creative, and in a school system where class sizes keep growing and children are not able to express themselves in their unique way, their learning and performance tends to get stifled.

Once again, a balanced approach of foundational aspects of psychological therapy, sound nutrition, hormonal, and pharmacological treatment if needed would be an optimal approach. Where you will see arguments on both sides that stimulants might protect the brain vs. causing a 'rewiring,' the fact is that these pharmaceuticals reduce the overall blood flow to the brain and disturb glucose metabolism.

So when we resort to prescribing a medication, this does not come without risks or consequences, and by ignoring the underlying causes, we are only putting on a temporary bandage allowing the real problem to grow and grow over time.

Nutritional Support

In addition to some of the foundational nutrients for depression such as B vitamins and Essential Fatty Acids, below are some common nutrients used to directly enhance ones mood as well as conditions of ADD and ADHD. Always consult a health care practitioner especially if you are on other medication therapies due to the fact you can get an overstimulation of neurotransmitters such as serotonin when antidepressant medications and supplements are combined.

In addition, only use high quality pharmaceutical grade supplements to avoid issues of contaminated products, toxic tagalongs, and to ensure you are getting the proper dosage of ingredients.

Mood Enhancement Natural Supplements include: 5-HTP (5 Hydroxy-tryptophan), Phosphatidylcholine, Phosphatidylserine, Inositol, St. Johns Wort, Tyrptophan and Tyrosine.

Supplements to support issues of ADD and ADHD include: EPA/DHA (Fish oils), American ginseng, Carnitine, 5-HTP (5 Hydroxy-tryptophan), Ginkgo Biloba, Magnesium, Phosphatidylserine, St. Johns Wort, L-Theanine.

Checklist for Mood and Behavior

1. Assess and address nutritional deficiencies from diet and from medication therapy.

2. Assess and address dietary food intolerances.

3. Diet. Refer to the chapter 7 for the backbone of a healthy diet, and when speaking of mood and behavior it is important to limit the amount of refined foods, sugars, flours, caffeine, artificial flavorings, colorings, preservatives and GMO's.

4. Healthy balance of relaxation techniques and exercise.

5. Supplements. Incorporating a combination of foundational nutrition as well as targeted supplements can serve someone very well. As you can see from above there are many options and an experienced practitioner can help dial in your needs. I do find that foundational nutrition of a quality and hypoallergenic multivitamin, EPA/DHA, probiotics, and phosphatidylserine can be of great benefit.

See also; Sleep, Thyroid, Food Intolerances, Adrenals and Stress, and Hormonal health and support.

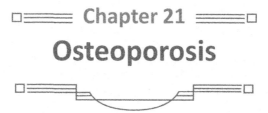

Chapter 21

Osteoporosis

Osteoporosis is a progressive disease where one's bones become porous and brittle, leaving them with a great susceptibility to bone fractures. It is estimated that by the age of 60, almost one-half of the women in the United States will have osteoporosis. One in five women will break a hip in their lifetime and one-half of the women who fall and break a hip will remain debilitated and never walk again. Aside from debilitation, hip fractures increase many other issues of morbidity.

According to the World Health Organization (WHO), osteoporosis is the second leading health care problem in the world, afflicting more than 200 million people. In the United States, osteoporosis is the cause of approximately 1.2 million cases of broken bones each year. Osteoporosis is not a gender specific disease, although where 1/3 cases involve men, the vast majority of cases of osteoporosis occur in post-menopausal women. This might lead to someone thinking that it is a hormone related disorder, and yes, that is partly correct.

Much of the formula of bone health resides around mineralization of the bone structure and what are known as osteoclasts and osteoblasts. To maintain your bone health, your body needs calcium, magnesium, boron, and vitamins D and K, so as you can see its more than just calcium as is mainly promoted in the realm of bone health.

Bone is a living, dynamic organism which works in a balance of building new healthy bone, and breaking down and getting rid of old and unhealthy, also known as resorption. What controls this balance are cells known as osteoclasts and osteoblasts. When resorption, or removal of old bone tissue by the osteoclasts occurs at a faster rate than synthesis of new tissue, bone health is then compromised.

Osteoclasts will break down old and unhealthy bone allowing for the formation of new bone. Osteoclasts actually break down the mineralization which results in a transfer of calcium and other parts of the bone matrix from bone fluid to the blood.

Osteoblasts are responsible for bone mineralization and bone formation. Osteoblasts decrease with age and they secrete what is known as osteocalcin which plays a significant role in bone mineralization and formation.

Calcitonin is a hormone which also plays a role in mineralization of bone. Calcitonin works to reduce blood calcium opposing the effects of parathyroid hormone which increases calcium in the blood. When working in optimal balance, healthy calcium mineralization is available for the bone structure.

Medications

Osteoporosis has led to a very healthy prescription market of drugs targeting prevention and even treatment, although as you will see, is not the only answer and one must look deeper to the reasons why our society is becoming so bone brittle. Balancing the condition of osteoporosis with choices of medication and/or nutrition often falls into a risk vs. benefit deal, which is why we will be looking at the causative factors and what people need to do for prevention.

There are various classes of drugs available for osteoporosis most involving the anti-resorptive agents such as bisphosphonates, estrogen therapy, SERMs (Selective Estrogen Receptor Modulators), and calcitonin.

Bisphosphonates represents the most widely used therapeutic class in the treatment of osteoporosis. These are oral drugs such as Fosamax, and Actonel as well as other infusion or injection type medications. One might argue their progression has been based off of convenience of dosage and not as much on efficacy as we have gone from a once daily tablet, to a once weekly, once monthly, and now there are infusions offered at just once to twice a year. This all sounds great, but let's take a look at some major side-effects of the bisphosphonate group of drugs.

Although widely in demand, these drugs possess significant drawbacks, either in the form of safety or efficacy. Where these drugs are indicated for the prevention of bone breaks due to excessive bone weakening and loss seen in osteoporosis, there have been some reports where they could actually lead to bone fractures, especially in the femur bones of people taking them for a number of years.

This should not be ultimately surprising considering the way that they work as anti-resorptive agents. Remember previously where we spoke about the purpose of resorption is to break down and get rid of old, unhealthy bone. So the reason these drugs might show a reduction in bone density is because they are keeping the old, unhealthy bone around which the body naturally would be getting rid of.

In fact, in 2010, the FDA confirmed that bisphosphonate drugs for osteoporosis carried a small, but meaningful risk of femoral fractures and ordered an update to product labels. Now we are seeing more recent research linking bisphosphonates to a higher chance of femur fractures.

Calcitonin salmon has been on the market and approved for treatment of osteoporosis since the 1970's. Calcitonin salmon (Miacalcin and Fortical) is inhaled, taken in pill form, or even injected. Miacalcin and Fortical are synthetic versions of calcitonin salmon, a hormone found in the bodies of mammals, birds, and fish. Although, as we have seen many times what is good for an animal is not necessarily good for a human, which appears to be true in this case as well.

The theory is that the synthetic version of salmon calcitonin should work like human calcitonin in keeping calcium out of the blood stream and into the bone structure, thus supporting bone structure. This must be how it has been approved by the FDA, right? Well, recent news is showing that this might not be the case, and not only may it not support bone structure, it might come with some other unwarranted side-effects.

FDA panelist Amy Whitaker has said "no studies have definitely shown that higher density actually reduces bone fractures," and calcitonin salmon "…has very little evidence of efficacy."

The FDA panel has recently voted that the risks of calcitonin salmon outweigh any benefits when used to treat osteoporosis. These risks you ask? Health authorities around the world have been reviewing the drug's safety after two recent studies showed a slightly higher rate of cancer among patients taking calcitonin pills.

SERMs (Selective Estrogen Receptor Modulators) have gained increase use over the years, but once again, not without risks. SERMs are designed to selectively work on the receptor to estrogenic actions on bone and anti-estrogenic actions on the uterus and breast. The problem is that these drugs tend to work differently in other tissues and parts of the body. The most common of these drugs is known as Evista® (raloxifine) which now comes with a warning of increased chance of developing blood clots, not something someone should take lightly.

What about the role that your body's natural hormones play? As we age our bodies decrease in their production of certain hormones, such as with a woman going through menopause and a man through andropause. Hormones such as estrogen, progesterone, testosterone and cortisol play a role in bone health, and this can be a major factor to the increase cases of osteoporosis in both women in men as they go through their changes in life, especially since we are becoming hormonally exhausted and imbalanced at an earlier age.

Testosterone, the 'male hormone,' plays a role in the bone health of both men and women in that it decreases bone deterioration and helps maintain bone strength. As both men and women enter into andropause and menopause respectively, their bodies lose the ability to create adequate amounts of testosterone. It's the same story with women in regards to progesterone and estrogen, so they get a double whammy as their ovaries stop producing estrogen and progesterone as they transition into menopause. Estrogen and Progesterone play roles in how they body builds new bone and gets rid of old bone, thus when hormonal imbalance occurs so does the balance of how the body builds new bone and rids itself of old bone.

Cortisol can be elevated due to mismanaged stress, this is a bone crusher. Cortisol being elevated consistently for a long period of time can attribute to bone matrix break down. Think about one of the major side-effects of steroid medication such as prednisone and why doctors don't like to keep people on these medications too long or too many times- brittle bones and increase chance of fracture. Thus if your natural cortisol remains high it can have the same effect.

The balance of hormones influence the activity and balance of osteoclasts and osteoblasts mentioned above, thus assessing ones hormonal balance including cortisol, sex hormones and even thyroid and restoring to appropriate levels may support the body's bone health.

Diet and Lifestyle Factors That Can Lead To Osteoporosis

Diet plays a very significant role in chances of someone getting osteoporosis. If the body does not get enough critical bone healthy nutrients such as calcium and magnesium, it will rob these essential minerals from the bones. Excessive intake of protein, salt, sugar, caffeine and carbonated soft drinks can be a problem as well. The effect that the foods you eat on pH also play a significant role. If you eat predominately acidifying foods (meats, sugar, dairy, etc.) and do not balance off with alkalinizing foods (herbs, vegetables, fruits), this can lead to an acidic pH in the blood stream, thus ushering in loss of bone minerals. Minerals are alkalinizing, so the body will monitor the blood stream and if too acidic will pull minerals such as calcium and magnesium out of the bones to acidify the blood stream. Lifestyle issues include smoking and alcohol consumption.

Avoid dairy. I know, this might sound contradictory to what you have heard and learn, but the truth be told, avoiding dairy is probably one of the best thing you can do for healthy bones. The assumption is that since dairy is high in calcium, it must be good for bones. The recommendation of dairy to be consumed via the U.S. government food plate and previous food pyramid is not based on science. More than likely, it's recommended based on the dairy industry interest and influence.

In fact, Harvard School of Public Health modified the U.S. Food Plate and designed their Healthy Eating Plate, omitting dairy. This should be of no surprise as Dr. Walter Wilett, one of the most cited researchers and chair of Nutrition at Harvard School of Public Health, has been instrumental in the development of the Healthy Eating Plate and a critic of the previous FDA Food Pyramid calling it "udderly" ridiculous. Dr. Willett purposely misspelled the word "utterly" in a report criticizing the food pyramid to emphasize the fact that the guidelines aren't based on scientific fact or key findings regarding health, most especially when it comes to dairy products, which have no evidence of being healthy for human consumption at all.

From an evolutionary point of view, dairy is a strange food for human consumption, it's great for a calf, but not for a human being. It is estimated that 75% of the world population is lactose (milk sugar) intolerant, and this is what has spurred an industry of dairy digestive foods and products.

The dairy industry has overstepped its boundaries in how it promotes the benefits of milk and dairy. You know the commercials with the milk mustaches, often using a celebrity or an athlete? The FTC has put a halt to a number of these ads due to a litany of claims not backed by scientific research such as benefiting sports performance, creating strong bones, losing weight and lowering high blood pressure.

Aside from the fact that the countries with the lowest dairy consumptions have the lowest rates of osteoporosis, there have been studies to back this up. The Harvard Nurses' Health Study reported in 1997 that, among 78,000 women followed for 12 years, those who got the most calcium from dairy products had approximately double the hip fracture rate, compared to women who got little or no calcium from dairy products. The July 2000 issue of *Pediatrics* similarly reports that, among girls 12 to 18, calcium intake had no effect on bone density, although exercise did help build strong bones.

Exercise

As far as exercise is concerned, weight bearing exercise is the best option for building bone. This means running, jumping, soccer, basketball, even dance will exercise the bone and support its growth better than non-weight bearing exercise such as swimming where gravity does not play a significant role. As always, gauge your level and type of exercise with your medical practitioner.

Supplementation

Nutritional supplementation offers great benefits for healthy bones, and it's not just about calcium. In fact, it's becoming more apparent that vitamin D might in fact play a larger role in bone health than calcium, although let's take a look at some of our favorite supplements for optimal bone health. Below I will list some of the most critical supplements in helping to support bone density and health.

Calcium- Calcium is a major component of the bone mineral matrix. Optimally use a source of high absorption such as a calcium hydroxyapatite or calcium citrate, opposed to the common over the counter calcium carbonate.

Magnesium- Magnesium is another major component of the bone mineral complex. Magnesium actually has over 300 roles in the body, thus important for other reasons in addition to bone health. Highly absorbable forms of magnesium include magnesium glycinate, aspartate, malate, or citrate, where the common over the counter magnesium chloride and oxide have much lower levels of absorption.

Vitamin D- Vitamin D promotes intestinal calcium and phosphorus absorption and reduces urinary calcium loss. Optimally one would have their active vitamin D levels tested with a goal of 25-OH D levels to be between 40 to 60 ng/dl. Vitamin D3 (cholecalciferol) is the preferred source over vitamin D2 (ergocalciferol), the common prescription form, as it has shown better absorption.

Vitamin K- Vitamin K enhances bone formation by enabling osteocalcin (hormone secreted by osteoblasts) to bind to calcium and promote healthy bone mineralization.

Ipriflavone- Ipriflavone helps to promote healthy bone balance a few different ways. Ipriflavone supports healthy collagen and formation of the bone mineral complex. Ipriflavone has also shown to promote the body's natural calcitonin which is critical in maintaining healthy intracellular calcium.

Strontium- Strontium is a trace mineral which supports collagen formation and osteoblast (bone building) activity. One thing to keep in mind is that strontium and calcium should not be taking together, since strontium is absorbed via the same transport mechanisms as calcium.

Checklist for Healthy Bone Support

1. **Diet.** Refer to the chapter 7 for the backbone of a healthy diet, and when speaking of healthy bones it is important to limit the amount of refined foods, sugars, flours and caffeine laden foods. Incorporate whole foods, fruits, vegetables and lean and clean proteins. Consider the elimination of dairy as well.

2. **Exercise.** For healthy bone building, weight baring exercises are important. See your practitioner on the best options to help provide healthy bone building and remodeling.

3. **Supplements.** I like to keep it simple. For maintenance I like to recommend Pure Encapsulations Cal/Mag with Co Factors. For advanced bone issues such as osteoporosis, I like to add strontium to the program to go towards a complete bone building complex with strontium such as Pro-Bono from OrthoMolecular.

   See also; adrenal and stress, hormonal balance and support.

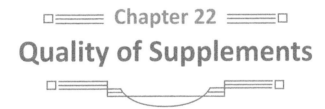

Chapter 22

Quality of Supplements

I have spoken a lot about nutritional supplementation since I feel is perfect alternative or complementary form of medicine. One thing I have to impress is upon quality of nutritional supplements. The fact is that there is a lot of junk on the market, often sold on a low price and volume for profit model, or sold behind a high dollar predatory marketing model.

The truth is there are very few regulations for nutritional supplements, and where I am not asking for more regulation of the industry, I do recommend supporting nutritional companies with the highest integrity. There are constant examples of supplements being contaminated or not having what they save they have in them. I will have a list of some of my favorites in the resource section, although there are many others, so below I will list some of the factors I look for to find a quality nutritional company.

Issues such as bioavailability (how much nutrient is actually available), manufacturing process, sourcing of quality nutrients which must be free of toxin's such as heavy metals and bacteria, not only contribute to nutritional deficiencies, but introduce a host of other problems as well.

Here are some factors I look for in a quality nutritional supplement:

- Free of common allergens and toxins such as: wheat, gluten, nuts, egg, soy, dairy, preservatives, hydrogenated oils, coatings, shellac, binders, fillers, excipients, sugars, artificial flavors, sweeteners and colorings.

- Vegetarian and non-porcine capsules to limit allergic reactions and toxin exposure.

- Ingredients sourced from trusted industry leaders and suppliers.

- Ingredients and raw materials tested for purity and potency by independent certified laboratories.

- Manufactured by a NSF and GMP registered laboratory which exceeds the standards of the United States Pharmacopeia (USP).

- Full disclosure- Supplement labels to list all ingredients, including composition of raw material as well as standardizations of herbal extracts provide to indicate primary active marker compounds.

- Transparency- A nutritional company who provides C of A's (Certificates of Analysis), and other documents to ensure quality and safety when asked for. I have seen too many companies who when asked for such documentation deny sharing it with the excuse of "proprietary information."

Check out _www.wholepharmacy.com_ for some of our favorite nutritional companies.

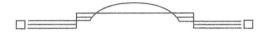

Part III:

TOOL BOX AND RESOURCES

So far I have given you the fundamentals, the ground work to move forward regardless of your state of health, or current life condition. The following are some of the many beneficial alternatives or complementary modalities one can use to support their lives.

These tools are different and varied; they extend the mind-body-spirit continuum and can be used in all areas of your life, not just health. After all, many issues of our health have stemmed from other areas of our life; relationships, money, stress, etc. so addressing these other issues with these tools can provide great benefit for one's health and overall wellbeing.

These are not the end all, there are obviously other modalities of healing and support to your healthy living, although one major area I think our health care system continually drives away from is self-care. For instance, I am a tremendous fan of chiropractic care and acupuncture, I feel they both, and others, offer tremendous benefits for our health and wellbeing. What I want to offer you here are tools and strategies in the spirit of self-care which you can choose to do in the comfort of your own home, or in a public class.

And understand, it takes commitment, you might start on one particular path and witness some struggles, maybe your consistency will drop, and you might miss a day or two finding yourself out of the new healthy habits program you were trying to implement. Do not let this sabotage you! Get back on that horse, develop a habit of discipline and you will come through on the winning end.

Many of these tools are designed to make your health naturally stronger, thus acting as a prevention of disease or it can result in a faster healing process if you do happen to fall ill. You will see that I often tie in actual scientific research to show that there is a way out of this over-medicated society, thus leading to a tremendous savings in the financials of health and enhancement of wellness and vitality. This is a holistic approach to health, we welcome it all- it is never a one size fits all deal. Feel free to incorporate some or all of these tools, road test others, see what modalities and tools work best, and fit best into your life.

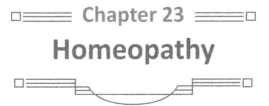

Chapter 23
Homeopathy

"The highest ideal of therapy is to restore health rapidly, gently, permanently; to remove and destroy the whole disease in the shortest, surest, least harmful way, according to clearly comprehensible principles."

-Samuel Hahnemann

When I was doing my clinical rounds for pharmacy at Hahnemann Hospital in Philadelphia, PA, curiously I never found much information on the teaching hospitals namesake…Samuel Hahnemann, the father of homeopathy. I understood that I was there for allopathic medicine, although even in 1994 I was searching for a more integrative approach and when I questioned my instructors if we would be learning anything in regards to homeopathy in the treatment of patient care, well, let's just say it fell on deaf ears.

Homeopathy is an exceptionally safe and effective form of medicine that treats the whole individual, is applicable to all ages, and is tremendously underutilized in the United States.

Through his work Hahnemann created some core practices to homeopathy which are now regularly practiced in integrative medicine, such as recognizing that one's health is the result of numerous forces acting on the human body including; genetics, environment, hygiene, stress (mental, emotional, physical), diet, and exercise. As you can see, Hahnemann was a man way before his time.

Samuel Hahnemann discovered homeopathy over 200 years ago with an experiment on himself, though perfectly healthy at the time, he found that by giving himself repeated doses of cinchona bark (quinine), he brought on all the symptoms of a malaria attack - fever with heat and chills. Quinine was a treatment for malaria.

Hahnemann then experimented by diluting then succussing a substance (shaking through striking the vial a number of times between numerical potencies). He realized that the potentised remedy was safer to use on the sick, unwanted side effects disappeared, and medicines were more effective.

Hahnemann tested 99 substances on himself and healthy volunteer's known as Provers, keeping detailed accounts of his observations, leading him to be the first practitioner to implement complete case taking in his patient assessments. He then matched the tested substances to heal symptoms of his patients using the Law of Similars.

Law of Similars or "like cures like," states that all pharmacologically active substances create a characteristic set of symptoms when administered to healthy people. It then recognizes that all sick people display a set of symptoms that are characteristic of their disease. The conclusion is then made that the cure may be obtained by administering weak/infinitesimal doses of substance whose experimental symptoms in healthy people are similar to symptoms displayed by the ill patient.

Due to the significance of dilution behind homeopathy, there is generally no fear of drug interactions, thus is safe to take in almost any situation, and often a suitable complement to prescription and nutrition therapy. Most homeopathic preparations are diluted down to the point where the active ingredients are no longer physically detectable.

The term homeopathy comes from two Greek words, *omia* (meaning "same"), and *pathos* (meaning "suffering"). What this means is that a homeopathic remedy is one that produces the same symptoms as those the sick person complains of, and in doing so sharply provokes the body into throwing them off.

Where the optimal choosing of a homeopathic medicine is based on a patient's mental, emotional and physical constitutional type as well as the totality of symptoms, let's take a look at some examples of homeopathic recommendations and ones symptoms based on the Law of Similars.

When someone has been stung by a bee they experience pain and inflammation, as well as a stinging feeling. A remedy for this can be Apis mellifica, the honey bee.

Another example is for people who have trouble sleeping. The homeopathic of coffee, coffee cruda, can be a remedy of choice.

A common one we use to help people alleviate hot flashes is Lachesis mutas. Lachesis mutas is the homeopathic of venom from the snake. What are the symptoms of a snake bite? Hot, burning, constricted feeling, just like a hot flash.

It is important to note that homeopathic preparations can be either over the counter or by prescription only.

Due to the fact that homeopathic remedies are closely controlled under the FDA, homeopathic preparations can actually make claims as if what they can treat, the opposite of nutritional supplements. For example if you were to pick up a tube of arnica you would see on the side that it says "Trauma, Bruises, and Muscle Soreness."

To hone in a step further, to make it easier to recommend homeopathic preparations, you can purchase what is known as a repertory. A repertory is an index of symptoms and systems of the body with remedies that affect the system listed under each heading.

For example, if I was to look up "Bronchitis," I would look for the exact symptoms the individual is experiencing. I dial into a symptom description that parallels that of the individuals such as "as symptoms get worse lying down or in stuffy rooms, cough is dry at night but loose in morning, lack of thirst." The remedy points to pulsatilla 6c.

Like nutrition, homeopathy is actually core to the practice of pharmacy. Most pharmacists in the 1800's and early 1900's were trained in compounding homeopathic/eclectic medicines.

Where homeopathy all but died out in the U.S. in the early 1900's it has been on a strong rebound in recent years. In the United States, of the people who try homeopathic agents, 84% say they would use them again.

In other countries through Europe homeopathy is the leading "alternative" treatment by physicians with growing numbers in the citizenry, and even taught in medical schools. And despite homeopathy's impressive popularity in Europe, it is actually even more popular in India where over 100 million people depend solely on this form of medical care.

In Switzerland, homeopathy has made such an impact that the government decided to study its efficacy and cost effectiveness. Despite the impressive technological prowess of conventional medicine today, the Swiss government has determined that homeopathy is considerably more cost effective.

The Swiss' "Health Technology Assessment" was a thorough analysis of a wide variety of clinical studies and laboratory research. The report also reviewed the body of evidence on cost-effectiveness research for homeopathic care, and it even conducted its own cost-effectiveness study among Swiss physicians and patients. The Swiss report found that total practice costs for physicians who specialized in homeopathic medicine had an overall 15.4 percent reduction in overall health care costs associated with their practice, as compared with physicians who practiced conventional medicine as well as those physicians who practice other "complementary and alternative medicine" treatments (but not homeopathic medicine.)

Homeopathy has a bright future in America, as it is the perfect complementary therapy to allopathic medicine and nutrition alike. Homeopathy has no known side-effects or interaction's, can be used by any age group, even animals, and is very inexpensive, while paralleling the growing trend of individualized medicine. Homeopathy can also be used in self-care, or one can seek out the expertise of a homeopathic practitioner.

□═══ **Chapter 24** ═══□

Meditation over Medication

"If we could bottle the benefits of meditation it would be a multimillion dollar drug."

- Frank Lipman MD

Meditation is one of the most powerful techniques and strategies that you can use for your health and wellbeing. It's easy, cheap, feels great, and comes with profound benefits. Meditation can be as easy as finding a quiet place while doing some breathing exercises, repeating a mantra or even incorporating visualization techniques and even physical exercise. And with the ease and advent of iPods and cellular phones you can download countless meditation apps for those who need a helping hand to get rolling.

Meditation is about stepping back from being lost in random, incessant thoughts. In fact a Harvard study shown that the average person is lost in thought about 47% of the time. Meditation is seeing thought and witnessing it without judgment, and with a relaxed mind. When you give yourself the chance to step back, you gain a different perspective; you familiarize yourself with the present moment *(not living in the past or the future.)* Meditation invites our minds to be our allies and we will become more open to break-through thinking- raising expectations and finding creative solutions. A regular meditation practice will promote focus, calmness, and clarity- who can't use more of that?

Meditation should be a regular practice, done daily. Meditation is all about you; it's your time so make sure you give yourself this, it can be done in as little as ten minutes a day. Like any new habit to create, such as exercise, research shows it takes 21 days to create a new habit. Many Yogis' will suggest a 40 day regimen, 40 straight days, feeling this is the length to make an impact, and that this is the length to make sure that your new habit sticks. I have seen too many people make it to the 21 day mark and fall off, whether it's a diet or exercise program, almost as if their goal was to go 21 days. This is why I recommend the 40 day yardstick, as by this point it becomes embedded into your daily routine.

A challenge I hear a lot about people getting into meditation is that they get distracted. Getting distracted during meditation is totally and completely natural. As you notice that you are lost in thought, step back from out from that thought and relax back into the present moment and experiencing being "here." Using a mantra or even an affirmation during a meditation can help with this greatly, you see yourself veering, mentally or vocally repeat your chosen mantra. A mantra is an energy based word or sound which is repeated aid concentration in meditation. The definition of 'mantra' is essentially to 'free your mind.' In Sanskrit, 'man' means 'mind', and 'tra' means 'freeing.' Remember in chapter 19 on memory and cognition when I spoke about the Kirtan Kriya? This is a singing exercise or meditation which uses the mantra or sounds of Saa Taa Naa Maa along with the repetitive finger movements.

You might have heard of the word or sound Om. Om is a Sanskrit sound from Hindu origin which is believed to be the first primordial sound of the Universe. There is a Tibetan mantra which you might have heard of which has been chanted universally for world peace which uses Om- *Om Mani Padme Hum.*

Affirmations are a great option and you can easily make them up or customize them to help guide your medication. You can look at an affirmation as a centering thought to help guide the intention of your meditation has well. Here are some examples of some mantras which you can repeat related to empowering your health:

"I create my perfect health"

"I live my life in balance"

"I live my life through creativity, passion and enthusiasm"

"I am a perfect expression of nature"

"I am perfect as I am"

"I choose foods that fill me with energy and help me thrive"

"I am flexible, powerful and balanced"

"I intend to take steps each day toward perfect health"

Meditation has been proven in numerous studies and outcome based situations to provide health related benefits including:

- Reduce pain
- Enhance the body's immune system
- Reduces feelings of depression, anxiety, anger and confusion
- Increases blood flow and slows the heart rate
- Provides a sense of calm, peace and balance
- Helps reverse heart disease
- Helps control thoughts
- Increase energy
- Reduces stress

Plus, let's talk about health care costs. There are numerous studies which point to a dramatic savings in health care costs, a major issue in our society, so let's take a look at a few of them.

- According to a study published in the *American Journal of Health Promotion* in 2011, people with consistently high healthcare costs experienced a 28% cumulative decrease in physician fees after an average five-year period practicing the Transcendental Meditation techniques compared with their baseline.

- According to a study published in *Psychosomatic Medicine* in 1987, a large study of the insurance statistics of 2,000 Transcendental Meditation participants over a 5-year period indicates what could happen if Transcendental Meditation were incorporated into existing health care programs. The study found that the Transcendental Meditation group had 55% less medical care utilization, both in-patient and out-patient, compared to controls matched for age, gender, and occupation. The Transcendental Meditation group had lower sickness rates in all categories of disease, including 87% less hospitalization for heart disease and 55% less for cancer.

- According to a study published in the *Journal of Social Behavior and Personality* in 2005, a study of Transcendental Meditation participants over the age of 65 investigated whether the Transcendental Meditation technique can reduce medical expenditures in the elderly. Payments to physicians for treating 163 Transcendental Meditation practitioners over the age of 65 were compared with those for 163 control subjects matched for age, sex and other factors. The TM group's five-year cumulative reduction in payments to physicians was 70% less than the control groups.

- According to the *American Journal of Hypertension* in 2005, several randomized studies indicate that the Transcendental Meditation technique reduces hypertension as effectively as drug therapies. In a study published in the *American Journal of Health Promotion* in 1996, the cost-effectiveness of the Transcendental Meditation technique was compared with the five leading anti-hypertension drugs over a period of 20 years. The study indicated that TM technique had the lowest cost and the most health benefits. The cost reduction of Transcendental Meditation ranged from 23.7% to 72.9% less than the anti-hypertensive medications.

Mindfulness over Mindlessness

Mindfulness in itself is a meditation which you can incorporate in every part of your daily life.

> *Mindfulness is a kind of energy that helps us to be aware of what is going on. Everyone is capable of being mindful. Those of us who practice daily have a greater capacity for being mindful than those who do not. Those who do not practice still have the seed of mindfulness, but its energy is very weak. By practicing just three days, the energy of mindfulness will already increase.*

> -Thich Nhat Hanh

It seems especially now in our culture, many of us are constantly running. We might not have yet gotten to where we want to be, and we keep running to get there while at the same time ignoring the present state as well as our own happiness. By being mindful of what is going on in the here and now, you have the chance to realize that there are plenty of conditions right in front of you to be happy.

It sounds almost too simplistic, but it's very real. Mindfulness is the capacity to recognize what's right in front of you, and to be aware of what is going on. The object of mindfulness can be anything; the blue sky, a cloud, birds, plants, the glass of wine in your hand, people around you. There can be mindfulness in everything you do; eating, drinking, walking, - even just looking at what's around you.

While you are drinking a cup of water, if you know that you are drinking water in that moment and you are not thinking of anything else, you are drinking mindfully. While you are walking, focus all your attention on the act of walking, you are walking mindfully. By doing this, you will begin to walk in such a way that every step brings you confidence, a sense of ease and freedom. Look up at the sky, what do you see? If it's a bright blue sky, recognize it as that; be aware of the beauty of the sky. Regardless of what the object is, you will begin to find a sense of calmness in the simplicity of mindfulness.

Mindfulness is the opposite of mindlessness which has become so rampant in our society with the increase in cellphones and other tools of technology. It seems we are always 'connected' and practically deny ourselves times of calmness and peace. How many times have you seen someone walking through a parking or sidewalk, controlled by Facebook updates on their cellphone or worst yet, while driving? This type of mindlessness only separates you from your true self, shuns peace, and invites in a disconnectedness type of chaos.

As you can see, this meditation thing is the real deal, so don't you think it's worth implementing this into your life? And besides all the benefits mentioned above, it feels great.

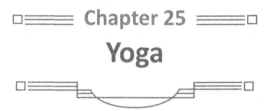

Chapter 25

Yoga

"Yoga teaches us to cure what need not be endured and endure what cannot be cured."

-B.K.S. Iyengar

If the history of Yoga in the U.S. is any sign of where we could be seeing complementary and lifestyle medicine going, we are looking at a bright future of health and wellness in our society. Think about it. Even though Hindu monks brought yoga to the West in the late 19th century, you started hearing about yoga as it gained steam in the late 60's and 70's and for many it still seemed like it was far out, something only hippies and the spiritual folk do. And now there are over 11 million regularly practicing yoga in the U.S., and you are likely to find numerous yoga studios and health clubs offering classes in your home town.

Do you know what I love about yoga? Anyone can learn yoga and there are a plethora of yoga classes to meet someone's need, whether they are a total beginner or advanced. Yoga is for everyone. There are so many different types, you can try and learn a new type of yoga constantly, never getting board, constantly growing, finding what type of yoga works best for you. Most fitness clubs, YMCA's offer yoga, and most likely you can find yoga studies right in your home town. There are plenty of Yoga DVD's and course on the internet to get you up and running in the comfort of your own home.

Yoga is a physical, mental, and spiritual discipline which, including breath control, simple meditation, and the adoption of specific bodily postures, is widely practiced for health and relaxation. Yoga originated in ancient India and has been practiced for over 5000 years and has a very strong track record from everything from increasing strength, balance, relaxation, reducing stress, and increased muscle tone.

So, let's take a look at some of the health benefits which have been backed up by research.

As you will see, much of yoga's benefits will be related to its ability to promote relaxation, although let's take a look at a few of the disease states and conditions where it has shown to be beneficial.

There have been a number of studies which have shown the benefits of using yoga as a tool to combat hypertension. In one particular study, yoga was studied up against general relaxation methods to see if one would be more effective over the other. In this study, 34 hypertensive patients were assigned at random either to six weeks' treatment by yoga relaxation methods with bio-feedback or to placebo therapy (general relaxation). Both groups showed a reduction in blood-pressure (from 168/100 to 141/84 mm. Hg in the treated group and from 169/101 to 160/96 mm. Hg in the control group).

So we see that relaxation itself plays a role, although the difference with greater results in the yoga group was highly significant. Then the control group was trained in yoga relaxation, and their blood-pressure fell to that of the other group (now used as controls), showing that the results were not unique due to variability's in the study participants.

Yoga is also used successfully for many different types of pain disorders. Research has shown yoga to be beneficial for relief of osteoarthritis in hands where those who practiced yoga just once per week for 8 weeks, and after assessing pain, strength, motion, joint circumference, tenderness, and hand function using the Stanford Hand Assessment questionnaire, the yoga treated group improved significantly more than the control group in the amount of pain during activity, tenderness and finger range of motion.

Other research has shown the benefits of yoga with lower back pain, an extremely common affliction. Two groups of people suffering chronic low back pain (CLBP) were randomized to either an immediate yoga based intervention for one hour twice a week for 6 weeks, or to a control group with no treatment during the observation period but received later yoga training. Outcome and assessment measures included the forward reach (FR) and sit and reach (SR) tests. All participants completed Oswestry Disability Index (ODI) and Beck Depression Inventory (BDI) questionnaires. Functional measurement scores showed improved balance and flexibility and decreased disability and depression for the yoga group. What was particularly encouraging was the improvement in issues of depression which is not uncommon in patients with chronic pain of any sort.

Carpal tunnel syndrome is often a condition which leads to surgical intervention, or at least restriction of movement through splints as well as the use of anti-inflammatory medications. So researchers set out to see how yoga might benefit carpal tunnel syndrome by assigning two groups of subjects. One group received a yoga-based intervention consisting of 11 yoga postures designed for strengthening, stretching, and balancing each joint in the upper body along with relaxation given twice weekly for 8 weeks. Patients in the control group were offered a wrist splint to supplement their current treatment. Subjects in the yoga group had significant improvement in grip strength and pain reduction, and changes in grip strength and pain were not significant for control subjects, and it was found that a yoga-based regimen was more effective than wrist splinting or no treatment in relieving some symptoms and signs of carpal tunnel syndrome.

Fibromyalgia first came on the scene as a mystery disease, and patients often did not know where to go, especially being told it was "all in their head" from their practitioners. Although a mounting body of literature recommends that treatment for fibromyalgia (FM) encompass medications, exercise and improvement of coping skills. A randomized controlled trial was put together to evaluate the effects of a comprehensive yoga intervention on FM symptoms and coping. A sample of 53 female FM patients were randomized to the 8-week Yoga of Awareness program (gentle poses, meditation, breathing exercises, yoga-based coping instructions, group discussions) or to wait-listed standard care. Data were analyzed by intention to treat. At post-treatment, women assigned to the yoga program showed significantly greater improvements on standardized measures of FM symptoms and functioning, including pain, fatigue, and mood, acceptance, and other coping strategies.

Asthma is a condition which has increased dramatically over the last couple of decades. Some would argue its better techniques of assessment, and where prescription medication is often the first line therapy, researchers found that yoga can be supportive in issues of yoga as well. In one particular study, fifty-three patients with asthma underwent training for two weeks in an integrated set of yoga exercises, including breathing exercises, physical postures, breath slowing techniques, meditation, and a devotional session, and were told to practice these exercises for 65 minutes daily.

They were then compared with a control group of 53 patients with asthma matched for age, sex, and type and severity of asthma, who continued to take their usual drugs. There was a significantly greater improvement in the group who practiced yoga in the weekly number of attacks of asthma, scores for drug treatment, and peak flow rate. This study shows the efficacy of yoga in the long term management of bronchial asthma, but the physiological basis for this beneficial effect needs to be examined in more detail.

So as you can see, aside from general stress relief, relaxation, toning, strengthening and flexibility, yoga has shown many great benefits to people's health, often times above what conventional therapies have offered.

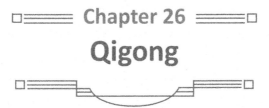

Chapter 26
Qigong

"*If you want to be healthy and live to one hundred, do qigong.*"

- Mehmet Oz

When we spoke about energy, we spoke about qi (chi), or life-force, and how one can work to support the flow of their life force energy, and how excess or deficient qi may result from disease, injury, or stress or energy blocks may then lead to further disease if not addressed.

Qigong (*pronounced chee gong*) is a practice of aligning breath, movement, and awareness for exercise, healing, and meditation. With a history dating back thousands of years and roots in Chinese medicine, martial arts, and philosophy, qigong is traditionally viewed as a practice to cultivate and balance qi or the flow of life-force energy. A qigong practice involves rhythmic breathing coordinated with slow stylized repetition of fluid movement, a calm mindful state, and visualization of guiding qi through the body.

The word qigong is a combination of two ideas. Qi is the vital energy of the body, and gong is the skill of working with the qi.

From a philosophical perspective qigong is believed to help develop human potential, allow access to higher realms of awareness, and awaken one's "true nature". From a health and medical perspective, in addition to Traditional Chinese Medicine, qigong has found its way into fields of integrative and alternative medicine and consists primarily of meditation, physical movements, and breathing exercises. Qigong can be practiced by an individual on oneself, as we are going to speak of here, as well as seeing a qigong master where they use the healing energy of qi on their patients.

Where qigong has been practiced for thousands of years, it was not until the 1980's when scientists in China began investigating the many medical benefits and claims in support of qigong. Below are some of the benefits which can be found in the literature as well as experienced by those who regularly practice qigong. As with any healing modality, it works best with an overall practice of wellness; including diet, mind, body, and spirit.

Qigong has shown benefits in studying its role in senile patients (combination of sitting mediation and gentle physical movements that emphasize a calm mind, relaxed body, and regular respiration). When qigong has been studied against regular exercises (walking, walking fast, or running slowly), qigong has produced greater improvement in areas of symptoms of senility, cerebral function, sexual function, serum lipid levels and function of endocrine (hormone) glands almost double the benefits that the general exercise group experienced. These results fall in line with other studies that have shown that dance helps memory, but the kicker is that one must continually learn new dances. So it's not just movement, its exercise and movement combined with mental stimulation.

Qigong has shown extensive benefits in regards to cardiovascular health. One particular study was done of hypertensive patients all on blood pressuring lowering medications. Half of the group practiced qigong for 30 minutes twice daily, and the other half did not practice qigong. The results show that the accumulated mortality (death) rate was 25.41% in the qigong group, and 40.8% in the non-qigong group.

The incidence of stroke was 20.5% in the qigong group and 40.7% in the non-qigong group, and the death rate due to stroke was 15.6% in the qigong group and 32.5% in the non-qigong group. The researchers also reported that over the initial 20 year period of the study, blood pressure of the qigong group stabilized, whereas that of the non-qigong group increased while drug dosages for the qigong group could be decreased and for 30% of the qigong group, discontinued. However the drug dosage for the non-qigong group had to be increased.

Cancer therapy has also seen an augmentation of success from qigong. In one particular study of cancer patients, qigong proved to be a valuable therapeutic aid for patients with advanced cancer. There were 97 patients who practiced qigong for more than 2 hours a day for 3 to 6 months, and 30 who did not practice qigong at all, all patients received drugs. Where both groups improved, the qigong group showed improvement in strength, appetite, freedom from diarrhea, and weight gain for to nine times greater than then the non-qigong group. Also the phagocytic rate, which is a measure of immune function, increased in the qigong group but decreased in the non-qigong group.

As you can see, qigong has proven to be a perfect complement to conventional drug therapy with benefits believed to stem from relaxation of the body, promotion of flow of qi (energy), blood, oxygen, and nutrients to all cells of the body, and promote removal of waste products from cells. It is no wonder that over 60 million people regularly practice qigong in China, and I believe if similar practices where employed in other nations, there would be dramatic changes to systems of health and disease.

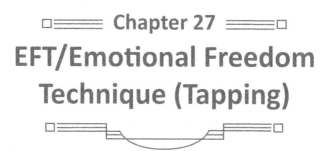

Chapter 27
EFT/Emotional Freedom Technique (Tapping)

Emotional Freedom Technique (EFT), or tapping, is a highly effective technique one can easily do wherever and whenever they want, and in relation to any situation that has an emotional charge to it. EFT is said to be used to clear personal blocks-emotional and energetic, and is used for improving health, attracting success, abundance, and overcoming challenges. I like to say it take the charge out of things.

Have you ever had a particular issue bugging you? It could be stirring up fear, worry, or any other negative emotion which keeps you off track, keeps you tense, and prevents you from working from your center. You are basically working on auto-drive of the ego. This is what EFT is great for.

As we spoke about earlier, every one of your thoughts, actions and vibrations create a quality of energy in your body, and either moves you towards your goals or away from your goals. Remember what Einstein said, your frequency needs to match the desires you want in order for you to get the results, and EFT is a tool to help align you with your desired vibration and frequency.

In order for you to attract what you want and move away from what you don't want, you need to (1) lower your emotional resistance or charge and (2) raise your vibration or frequency. We spoke about qigong as an ability to help move energy, or unblock energy in the system; EFT is another tool to help clear such blocks and is related to ancient Chinese medicine through acupressure and acupuncture points.

What we will do is share with you the basics of EFT, and give you examples of an EFT tap along sequence to lower your emotional resistance by clearing your mind and energy system of blocks. If you Google EFT you will find it's beneficial for all types of issues, from weight loss to migraines, to attracting abundance, improving relationships and more. This should be no surprise as we already spoke about how any condition, whether it relates to your health, relationships, finances, has an emotional element in its inception.

When you think about any issue you have, in regards to health, wealth or relationships, notice if there is an emotional charge involved. Even if there are events or issues in your life which are bringing down your vibration, these in fact can take a direct hit upon your health. Maybe you are stressed over finances, and you notice how your back then begins to stiffen up?

Maybe after a stressful time (such as the holidays), it seems you are running on adrenaline to make it through, but when the stressful time is over the "bottom falls out" and you get sick? Or it could be a flare up of an autoimmune condition, increased digestive problems, or stress leads to inability to cope and then depression? These are all examples where we can use a little help taking the energetic edge off, and EFT can help, so let's get started find out how to lower your emotional resistance and raise your vibration.

1. Step one is to focus on an emotional issue or block. It could be "frustrated at boss," "stressed about finances," or "worried about a loved one's health."

2. Next, start with a reference point of intensity in regards to the chosen emotional issue or block. Give it a level of intensity from 0 to 10 on how it affects how you feel. Zero meaning it has basically no emotional impact, and 10, off the charts, highly uncomfortable. So from a scale of 0 to 10, how anxious or upset does it make you feel, how true does the belief feel to you, or how intense is this discomfort.

3. Choose a set up statement. A set up statement is a statement which combines the emotional target or issue with a statement of acceptance. For instance, if a driving issue for stress in your life is dealing with a brother or sister in regards to a situation with your aging parents, then a target statement could be; "I experience stress and anxiety over dealing with mom and dad's situation with my sibling." Then we want to add this into a statement of acceptance, and this will be your set up statement. "Even though I experience stress and anxiety over dealing with mom and dad's situation with my siblings, I love and accept myself anyway."

Now we go through two different rounds, one is a Negative Tapping Sequence and the other is a Positive Tapping Sequence.

In the Negative Tapping Sequence, we tap on the sequence points while repeating the problem out loud. We can do this how every many times till we feel we have sufficiently taking the charge out of the situation. In the Positive Tapping Sequence, we tap on the sequence points while talking about possible solutions or positive outcomes for the target which you chose to identify and work on.

In a nutshell:

- Choose a target (emotion, limiting belief, health issue or symptom, or event)

- Rate the intensity

- Repeat the setup statement three times with the Karate Chop Point on the hand

- Perform negative tapping round sequence

- Perform Positive tapping round sequence

Example: #1 (follow along with the diagram for assistance on points of reference)

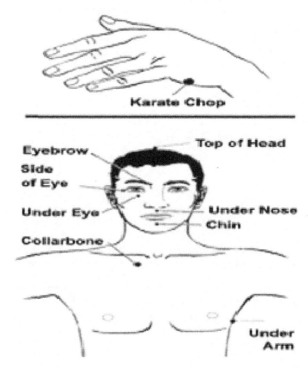

1. Karate Chop to the hand 3 times. "Even though I experience stress and anxiety over dealing with mom and dad's situation with my siblings, I love and accept myself anyway."

Now you will tap on the points of orientation 7 to 10 times while repeating the same or similar statements related to the negative issue.

2. Eyebrow point- "I am really stressed about mom and dad"

3. Side of eye- "I am worried that mom and dad are not being cared for"

4. Under Eye- "What's even more stressful is how my brothers and sisters are handling this"

5. Under nose- "I really don't think they have mom and dad's best interest at hand"

6. Chin-"This situation is taken its toll on me"

7. Collarbone- "It's no wonder I have trouble sleeping"

8. Under arm- "I don't see an easy solution to this problem"

9. Top of head- "This situation about mom and dad really has be worried"

Now, take a deep breath, and see how you feel. Measure your level of intensity, if it has not decreased, repeat steps 2 through 9, until you feel that release of intensity.

Positive affirmation cycle. Now you will tap on the points of orientation 7 to 10 times while repeating the same or similar statements related to a positive solution or perception of the problem.

1. Eyebrow point- "I know there is a solution to the problem with mom and dad"

2. Side of eye- "It might not be right in front of me, although I know that it's there"

3. Under Eye- "I understand my brothers and sisters are just as stressed as me, although we all have mom and dad's best interest in mind "

4. Under nose- "Sometimes it just takes a little communicating and everything will be all right"

5. Chin-"I understand that the answer is right around the corner, and I believe it's coming"

6. Collarbone- "Knowing the solution is on its way make me feel so much better"

7. Under arm- "And I know mom and dad are happy, and that's what really matters"

8. Top of head- "It feels wonderful to be free of the stress and anxiety relating to mom and dad"

9. Now, take a deep breath, measure the level of intensity again. How do you feel? Takes the edge off, right?

Example: #2 Let do an example on a health challenge, such as pain. I mentioned previously in most cases of pain, there is something called TMS (tension myositis syndrome,) which address the emotional link to the physical representation of pain.

1. Karate Chop to the hand 3 times. "Even though my neck and my shoulder has stiffened up and gone in to muscle spasms, I love and accept myself anyway." Now you will tap on the points of orientation 7 to 10 times while repeating the same or similar statements related to the negative issue.

2. Eyebrow point- "My neck is so stiff and it really hurts"

3. Side of eye- "It's just so frustrating because I have a lot to get done"

4. Under Eye- "The pain is zapping my energy and I don't feel motivated"

5. Under nose- "My neck really hurts; I don't know how I am going to get my work done"

6. Chin-"This situation is taken its toll on me"

7. Collarbone- "It hurts so much I can't even get a decent night's sleep"

8. Under arm- "Even the anti-inflammatories don't seem to be making a dent"

9. Top of head- "I haven't realized how much I rely on my neck and shoulders to be in healthy shape, this really is a drag"

Now, take a deep breath, and see how you feel. Measure your level of intensity, if it has not decreased, repeat steps 2 through 9, until you feel that release of intensity.

Positive affirmation cycle. Now you will tap on the points of orientation 7 to 10 times while repeating the same or similar statements related to a positive solution or perception of the problem.

1. Eyebrow point- "I know that my shoulders and my neck are only a temporary setback"

2. Side of eye- "In fact, I know it's a message that I need to slow down and chill out"

3. Under Eye- "My responsibilities will get done at the right time"

1. Under nose- "I realize that worrying will only make my pain worse"

2. Chin-"Just this realization already makes me feel better"

3. Collarbone- "I know the solution is on its way to make me feel so much better"

4. Under arm- "I felt good before, and I will feel good real soon"

5. Top of head- "It feels wonderful to realize that my neck and back are already healing"

Now, take a deep breath, measure the level of intensity again. How do you feel? Takes the edge off, right?

As I said you can use this for any problem with an emotional charge and there are a ton of resources, books, DVD, consulting, etc. from EFT instructors who can help you dial into your exact issues. You can get creative, create your own scripts or find one of the many products on the market that can hold your hand and walk you through it.

Give EFT a try, and I am confident you will see the charge taken out of almost any emotional issues, and feel the blocks dissolve away.

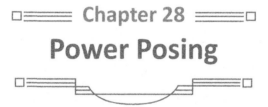

Chapter 28

Power Posing

I would like to suggest that you experiment with power posing. This is not just about health; in fact the studies on power posing are mostly based on the subject of high performance, building confidence, assertiveness, creativity and how one reacts in stressful situations. Although what has been seen in the studies is that in just 2 minutes, power posing can result in profound physiological changes which play a very large role in someone's health and wellbeing.

As I alluded to in chapter 6, Amy J.C. Cuddy, a social psychologist and professor at Harvard Business School, has shown that by tiny tweaks in your physical posture your body influences your mind patterns and beliefs, thus produce outwardly results in powerful ways.

The research on body language and non-verbal communication has mostly been based on the inference people make about us; how strong we appear to be, if we seem trust worthy, competent, how much someone might like us. This happens quickly, often within a few seconds and can have implications on an election outcome, who gets hired, who gets promoted, and who gets asked out on a date.

What the research has not delved into as much is how non-verbal behaviors influence who we feel about ourselves and how we inwardly and outwardly express this through our physiology; how confident, enthusiastic, authentic and comfortable we appear to be.

As a professor of MBA programs, Amy and colleagues have noticed that students who express themselves through high power non-verbal communication participated more in class. Those who participated more in class had a better chance to excel, thus there was a correlation between how someone expressed themselves with high power non-verbal communication and a greater opportunity to excel, over those who did not.

Power poses are non-verbal expressions of power and dominance. A high power pose is about taking up space, opening yourself up. A low power pose is about closing yourself inward, retracting yourself from the space that is around you. Below you will see a few examples of both.

Take a look at the power pose called "Pride." This is the pose you will often see a runner does when they cross the finish line first; hands raised

 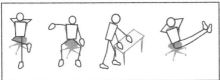 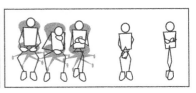

Pride   High Power Poses   Low Power Poses

and chin up. The interesting thing about this is that they have done studies of those who can see and those who have been blind since birth in how they react when winning or crossing the finish line first. The blind people react the exact same way in the "pride position," which shows this is not a learned experience, but an innate expression of pride and success.

One of my favorite breathing meditations which I learned from Garbrielle Bernstein is called "ego eradicator" which combines the pride power pose with a breathing technique called "breath of fire." After I learned about the science behind the "pride" power pose it made so much sense. If you remember how we spoke about ego and the negative influence it can have over us, the goal is not to be controlled by our ego- but to eradicate and overcome it. Would the true feeling of self-confidence, of pride and success not do this?

Through her research Amy Cuddy realized that high performance athletes, executives, leaders, even primates and animals, are more assertive, confident, and optimistic, they think more abstractly and take more risks. Since researchers have proven that when you are happy you smile, although if you are forced to smile by putting a pencil between your teeth, you also become happy even if you were not happy to begin with, Amy and her colleagues then went off to see if striking a power pose can make someone feel more powerful.

They based their studies on a few factors such as; ask participants how they felt, could striking a power pose make someone take more risks, and what would it do to their hormones, specifically testosterone and cortisol? Testosterone is the dominance hormone and cortisol is the stress hormone. As we spoke about in the chapter on hormones, the goal is to find a healthy balance of our hormones since our hormones are chemical messengers, hormones affect how we act and react, and the best leaders have higher testosterone and lower cortisol- this is across the evolutionary spectrum. The results of the study were amazing.

By partaking in high power poses for just 2 minutes, testosterone rose 20%, cortisol decreased 25%, and by partaking in low power poses, testosterone decreased 10% and cortisol rose 15%. Now, these studies were done by power posing for just 2 minutes, simple enough, we don't know is how long the hormonal change lasts. None the less, this is a very simple tweak with profound results of making you feel more powerful through physiological changes in your body.

This has implications for all levels of your being, from your health to efforts of high performance; here are just a few examples:

- At night time in hopes to bring down cortisol levels which when high can contribute to trouble sleeping.

- Use before any situation which might appear stressful; talking to your doctor, negotiations, a public speech, an interview.

Personally, I like to incorporate a 2 minute power pose to complete my morning meditation, and am conscious about implementing power poses throughout the day, whether I am sitting, standing or just relaxing.

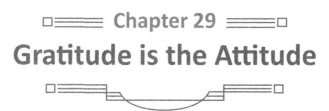

Chapter 29

Gratitude is the Attitude

"The attitude of gratitude is the highest yoga."

\- Yogi Bhajan

Gratitude is an amazing tool for all levels of your wellbeing, and as research has shown, your happiness. Think about it, what is our medicals system usual response or way to treat unhappiness? Anti-depressant medications, right? And we know there are mood and wellbeing benefits related to eating healthy, getting adequate sleep, stress management, and exercise. What many people do not know is that practicing gratitude is one of the most effective ways to shift and reset your happiness level.

Research has shown time and time again that people generally have a preset level of happiness. What this means is that regardless of a particular trauma or a highly positive outcome, peoples level of happiness generally tends to go back to its norm after about 3 months' time. One particular study took two groups of people; lottery winners and folks who through a physical trauma became paraplegics or quadriplegics. The participants in the study were monitored, and after 3 months' time, which group do you think was happier than before the particular event, winning the lottery or becoming crippled? The answer might surprise you- the results were equal. Each group found their way back to their set point of happiness, regardless of which life altering event they experienced.

Further studies have shown that happiness can be synthesized or artificially produced. This would fall in line with the mood elevation or high that shopaholics get from shopping, although as shown above in the example of winning the lottery, if the synthesizing effort exits the situation, then we go back to our normal set point. Since the chances of winning the lottery on a regular basis are slim, what if I was to tell you that by simply focusing on 5 things you are grateful for every week, you can raise continually keep yourself 25% happier and healthier?

Research on gratitude has shown to increase ones happiness by a full 25% which is actually better than the results antidepressant prescription drugs have shown in many studies. A particular study divided three groups of people. One group focused on 5 things they were grateful for every week, another group focused on 5 things that bothered them and caused them stress and anxiety, and the third group, 5 random events.

People who were in the gratitude group felt fully 25% happier than either of the other two groups; they were more optimistic about the future, managed stress better, they felt better about their lives and they even did almost 1.5 hours more exercise a week.

The types of things people listed in the grateful condition included:

- Sunset through the clouds.

- The chance to be alive.

- The generosity of friends.

And in the hassles conditions:

- Taxes.

- Hard to find parking.

- Burned my macaroni and cheese.

In Sonja Lyubomirsky's *The How of Happiness: A New Approach to Getting the Life You Want*, she refers to gratitude as "a kind of meta-strategy for achieving happiness." Lyubomirsky's research demonstrates that expressing gratitude has several benefits. People who are grateful are likely to be happier, hopeful and energetic, and they possess positive emotions more frequently. Individuals also tend to be more spiritual or religious, forgiving, empathetic and helpful, while being less depressed, envious or neurotic.

In addition, gratitude fosters happiness, making it easier to cope with stress and trauma. A positive perspective allows you to obtain a better grasp on suffering. "Expressing gratefulness during personal adversity like loss or chronic illness, as hard as that might be, can help you adjust, move on, and perhaps begin anew," Lyubomirsky says. In the days following September 11, 2001, gratitude was found to be the second most commonly held emotion (sympathy was the first).

Create Your Gratitude List

Think back and write out a list of five to ten persons, places, or things that you are grateful for. They can be big or very minute, as you saw above, something as simple as a sunset will do. Read them at least once a week, and especially in times when you are feeling a bit low. Remember, if you don't show appreciation or gratitude for what you have, the universe will not send you anymore gratitude.

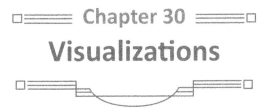

Chapter 30
Visualizations

Visualizations are a very powerful tool, and studies have shown that just by the act of visualizing a particular event or exercise, you stimulate the same areas of the brain as actually physically performing the event or exercise. For instance, one study took three groups of people and the goal was to improve their skills at shooting basketball free throws. The first group visualized shooting free throws without practicing, the second group physically practiced free throws, and the third group did neither. Groups one and two shown similar improvements and group three did not improve at all. So in this example, there was little difference between visualizing and practicing, while doing nothing shown no benefit at all.

Keep in mind; this is not an excuse not to take action if you really want to excel. Golfers and other pro athlete's use visualizing like a religion, while combining it with physical practice.

All this falls in line with the self-image we spoke about earlier. As part of your healing practice, consider a practice of visualizations. Basically, put a few minutes aside, take a few breaths to center yourself, and begin to visualize and feel what it would be like to live the life you would like to live. You can combine this with meditation, prayer, or any other practice or relaxation technique. Visualize any challenges or limitations of health to be gone. See yourself doing what you would love to be doing, with whom and where you would love to be doing it. Feel what it would feel like; allow the emotions to pour into and through you as if you were doing it.

As you can see visualizations are simple, they do not have to take long, and there are many techniques and programs that teach this in an enhanced form. Some other programs you might find value in are the Maxwell Maltz's Psycho-cybernetics, the Sylvan mind method, and numerous books and techniques based on NLP such as *NLP: The New Technology of Achievement*.

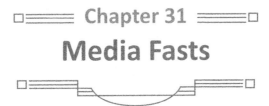

Chapter 31
Media Fasts

"We have become a world of people thinking the same thoughts at the same time." - Jack Kerouac

(Jack Kerouac's comment to the growing television generation of the 1950's)

Emotional and mental triggering through the media (and now social media) is an enormous influence in our society and your health and wellbeing. How often do you hear someone speaking out of fear about something they heard on the morning news, a political post shared on Facebook, a twitter rant? What a way to start the day.

There are many avenues that emotional triggering is delivered through the media: your television, radio, newspaper, magazine, cellphones and computer.

Wayne Dyer states in his book, *The Power of Intention*, "By the age of 14, the average child will have witnessed 12,000 murders in their own living room." If you think such a strong emotional charge witnessed 12,000 times over has no impact, think again.

News and media fasts are very important for the health of one's psyche. The bombardment of fear-based news is sometimes too much for the psyche to handle on both a conscious and subconscious level. Take a break from it. For a few days avoid all sources of news and media and see how you feel; take notes. Notice what goes through your head and compare with the thoughts that went through your head when you were an active news junkie. Notice if you feel a void. The separation from any pattern in life will present a void especially a pattern so strongly embedded. Fill that void with empowering thoughts from within, not the tactically manufactured thoughts from the external world.

Live your own story,
not someone else's.

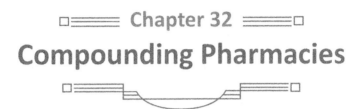

Chapter 32
Compounding Pharmacies

I owe a lot to the practice and the culture of pharmaceutical compounding. This is what gave me the ability to create a pharmacy which I believed in. This is where pharmacy got its roots, it's the art and the science of creating customized solutions for patient's needs.

Manufactured medications often only address people in a one size fits all approach. The reality is that millions of patients have unique health needs that off-the-shelf, manufactured medications cannot meet. For these patients, personalized medications prescribed by licensed practitioners and prepared by trained, licensed pharmacists offer a targeted solution for better health.

Working with a physician, a compounding pharmacist can meet individual needs of children, adults and animals. Whether it's an allergy to a dye or ingredient, a need for a different strength, customized natural hormonal therapy, or a preference for a different dosage form, compounding pharmacists provide patients with solutions to their medication needs.

What I really want you to understand is that the profession of pharmacy compounding has been under attack from Big Pharma as well as regulatory bodies, and I believe it is yet another attack on entrepreneurship, the engine behind the American economy.

I encourage you to check out _www.protectmycompounds.com_ which will offer more information on the benefits and the challenges the practice of compounding faces.

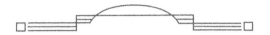

Part IV:

THE WHOLE
HEALTH
PRESCRIPTION

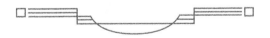

Here we are, and at this point you have had a lot of information thrown at you, spanning topics you might not have expected or quite frankly were not aware of. As you now know, health is multidimensional, health matters and it's important to incorporate a healthy and fun routine into your daily activities and lifestyle. This is about a healthy lifestyle approach, not just an eight week program. Healthy living does not have to be difficult, make health fun, and make it lively. Enjoy your exercise, savor some tasty and healthy foods, spend regular YOU time in quietness, enjoy time with loved ones, and understand that you can maintain, or even take your health back.

One of the last tips I would like to share with you is blue zones, because the people that live in these regions have figured something out. Blue zones are geographical locals where some of the oldest and healthiest people in the world live. These folks are the definition of adding years to their lives and life to their years. Researchers have discovered that these folks share certain traits, regardless of what country, region or climate.

- Staying active in mind and body
- Living with a sense of purpose
- Being around youth
- Socialization and connection to people

If You Can Take Away One Thing, Let It Be The Mind Body...

We talked a lot about the mind body, how ones thoughts and emotions can affect one's health. Sometimes it's as if we have to get out of our own way, although it's often easier said than done, and as we spoke about earlier, we can get caught up in egos projections and reactions which serve us no good. Here is a quick 3 step process in helping to heal your mind, emotions and take the fire out of them.

1. Be aware and recognize when you have a disempowering thought or emotion.

2. Forgive yourself when you find yourself caught up in the egos drama. Remember the quote from Gabrielle Bernstein? "*I forgive myself for having this thought- I choose love instead.*"

3. Shift your perception. Step back from the situation and ask yourself, is the ultimate truth what I perceive this to be? Offer yourself the ability to take a new perspective on the situation, a perspective that does not drain you, but strengthens you.

9 Simple Keys To The Whole Health Prescription

Below are 9 Simple Keys I would like to share with you, **The Whole Pharmacy Prescription**, which are simple steps to radical and lasting change towards a healthy path.

1. **Hydrate**- Start the day with a glass of pure, filtered water, and consume throughout the day. Our bodies become dehydrated through the night, so it is important to start the day by getting water back to our cells, especially before going for a caffeine related drink. One might want add the juice from a lemon- lemon has a way to help alkalinize your system. Clean water is critical; it would do your health wonders to invest in a home and even portable water purifying system. Quality water should have healthy minerals, although be free of other contaminants such as fluoride, chlorine, heavy metals, arsenic, and pathogens, while providing a water with an alkaline pH. These can be basic and economical or even on a grander whole house system. Check out _www.wholepharmacy.com_ for some of our favorite water purifying systems.

2. **YOU Time**- Finding quiet time for you is one of the most important things you can do, although in many cases seldom gets done. This is a time for meditation, introspection, prayer, however you want to spend it. Yogi and meditation masters call this "sadhana," which is devoted to self. You can call it what you want, although I encourage you to allow and give yourself this time every day.

"Any day you don't do sadhana, you have lost yourself to yourself. We do sadhana for our self so we can be clear headed and of clear conscious. When you don't do your sadhana – you blame circumstances."- Yogi Bhajan

Basically, starting the day with a time of quietness and meditation, you put your strong foot forward to not let your ego control you in the day ahead. And yes, the morning is best, get up just a few minutes early before your day begins to take hold, and YOU time gets pushed to the background.

Do not go to email, social media or anything else first- commit this time to yourself. And for just ten to fifteen minutes a day- anyone can do this. How much time do people find themselves mindlessly surfing Facebook or playing on their cellphone. The time is there, you just have to give it to yourself.

3. **Greens Drink/Smoothie**- What a great way to break the nighttime fast (break-fast) and get some nutritional density into your system. Whether you choose to blend your own fruit and vegetable drinks or purchase one of the high quality greens drinks on the market, you are starting the day with an alkalinizing food source, while providing your body with multiple servings of fruits and vegetables before the day even begins. One might also decide to add a scoop of a mineral complex, maybe a calcium and magnesium powder to the drink. As Linus Pauling has said, who was famous for his work with Vitamin C, *"The lack of minerals is the root of all disease."*

4. **Protein for Breakfast**- Starting the day with a healthy protein allows your body to begin the day working off of your energy creation cycle, and not over stimulating your pancreas and challenging your blood sugar with common breakfast foods such as grain only based meals. This can be the smoothie I mentioned above, adding protein from nuts, avocado's' or even complementing it with protein powder. You can have your wholegrain foods, but don't make it a grain only breakfast; in this case you can be putting too much stress on the pancreas and blood sugar. Make sure you have some healthy proteins and even fats with your meal. A protein shake by itself can

make it easier for you, and many come with foundational multivitamins and antioxidants on board.

5. **Honor your teeth and mouth**: Many people do not realize that the mouth can be a tremendous source of infections going systemic into the body. There is mounting evidence of how your teeth actually connect with meridian lines and organ systems through the body. When we do not regularly brush and floss, the result is that bacteria feed off plaque and get into the bloodstream, leading to heart disease and increasing your risk of stroke. Make it a point to give your mouth and teeth daily attention through flossing, brushing and tongue cleaning. As far as fluoride toothpaste, I am not a fan and recommend avoiding it, unless clearly needed and addressed by your dental professional.

6. **Healthy Diet and Foundational Nutrition**- A healthy diet should come as no surprise, and I eluded to diet numerous times previously in this book. One thing to keep in mind is portion size. Our culture has gradually gone down the "bigger the better" path which leads people consuming more calories than they actually need. Be conscious of portion size and try this trick. Be mindful of when you feel 80% full, and stop eating. Often times we keep eating until we feel full. By stopping when you are 80% full, this will allow your digestion to catch up to you and you will feel full without consuming the extra food, often unnecessary calories.

Depending on your food sources, how they have been grown, if pesticides have been used, how long they have been in transit and stored- they might not have the nutritional density one would hope for, thus foundational supplementation can be of benefit. The backbone to any foundational nutritional program should include:

- Comprehensive multivitamin
- Essential Fatty Acids (EFA/DHA)-ex-Fish Oil supplements
- Optimized vitamin D levels
- Probiotics

If you are on medications; be aware of the drug induced nutrient depletions we spoke of earlier. Talk to your pharmacist or grab your own copy of Jim LaValle and Ross Pelton's, *The Nutritional Cost of Drugs*, or Suzy Cohen's *Drug Mugger's*. Optimally you can have a proper nutritional assessment done from a qualified practitioner to dial in and assess your body's needs.

7. **Keep Moving Throughout the Day**- There is research to show that people who spend long hours sitting are at a greater risk of dying of serious illness, even if they eat healthy or work out. If you sit throughout the day, get up every 30 minutes to stretch out your limbs.

8. **Incorporate Exercise and Moving Meditation**- I shared with you some examples of moving meditation and how they can incorporated into an exercise program, such as yoga, qigong, and tai chi. Try some of these out, find out which ones vibe with you best. There are many options to do at home or you can go to a local studio or gym- and as you remember from above, they can come with some profound benefits to the health of the mind, body and spirit. Find a program which works best for you, incorporate a moving meditation other cardiovascular and weight bearing exercise programs- all based on your individual needs and current status of health.

9. **Incorporate Stress relieving techniques throughout day**- Remember how we spoke about how the body can adapt to stress throughout the day, by giving times of intense focus and work, and other times of rest and repair? The body goes through what are called ultradian rhythm's, which are mini cycles every couple of hours throughout the day- much like a circadian rhythm of day to night- awake to rest. Make sure you attend to times of rest and repair throughout the day, disconnect from the electronic OCD many people fall victim to.

   Consider taking some time to do some deep breathing, such as every 30 or 60 minutes, stop what you are doing and take 3 deep breaths. Breathing techniques allow you to oxygenate your body and cells, especially when under constant stress many people go through the day breathing very shallowly. Deep breathing will also provide instant relaxation taking you out of a stress cycle you might be in. And remember, breath right. On the in-breath, your diaphragm should extend out, on the out-breath, come back in.

Strike a pose! Remember power posing? All it takes is two minutes to incorporate a power pose, and be mindful of how you sit, stand and present yourself throughout the day; as you have seen, the results can be profound.

Well, it looks like our time is up. I really appreciate the time you took to check out my book, I hope that I have enlightened you to some realities of our medical system which I believe can be fixed. I encourage you to look us up at _www.wholepharmacy.com_ to keep up in the latest tips and strategies to add years to your life and life to your years. You will also find some of our favorite resources and strategies on how to live the very best and healthiest and empowered life for yourself.

In this book I wanted to offer options in self health care, ways you can begin to take back control of your health. I also want to share that there are many other medical modalities that often don't fall under the conventional paradigm which can be of great benefit as well, such as chiropractic care, acupuncture, medical massage and muscle testing _(my favorite being Quantum Reflex Analysis)_ through Premier Research Laboratories, and more. Thus understand there are many tools at your disposal.

I honestly believe we can turn this system around for the better, there is plenty of room for us all to be healthy and prosper, and change the path of our health and the health of our health care system.

Thanks,
Rob

Index

A

acid reflux   109, 223, 227-9
adaptogens   113-15, 117
adrenal fatigue   107, 109, 117-18, 122
adrenal glands   105-7, 112-13, 116, 133-4, 136, 138, 148, 172
adrenal support   115-16, 140, 146
aluminum   178, 201, 209-10, 222
Alzheimer   91, 93, 152, 176-8, 181-4, 188, 190, 203
Alzheimer's disease (AD)   9, 84, 86-8, 129, 152, 171-2, 174, 176-8, 180-8, 192, 209
Amyloid precursor protein (APP)   177, 184
andropause   125-7, 136-7, 247
asthma   41, 91, 93, 152, 211, 223, 270
autism   32, 84, 87, 91, 93, 208-9, 211, 223, 231-3

B

berberine   155-6, 158, 168, 170, 183-4
blood pressure   99, 111, 128, 157, 164, 166, 168-9, 195, 197-8, 205, 273
blood sugar   116, 152, 161-2, 166-9, 174, 297
breast cancer   37, 64, 83, 120, 131, 133, 135, 147
breathing exercises   112-13, 120, 261, 270, 272

C

cardiovascular disease   100, 152, 155-7, 181, 194-5
CDC (Centers for Disease Control)   39, 103, 209, 215-17, 239
cervical cancer   219-21
cholesterol   88, 99-100, 135, 137, 152, 154-6, 159, 163, 169-70, 194-5, 197, 237
chromium   155, 158, 169-70

CoEnzyme Q10   98, 156-8
cortisol   34, 67, 106, 113-14, 116, 135, 138, 141, 154, 172, 174, 186, 190, 247, 283
cortisol levels   113-14, 116, 121, 138, 172
crohn's disease   91, 93, 227
curcumin   157, 183, 185, 197, 221

D

dairy   82, 92, 94, 103, 205, 248-9, 251, 253
dementia   32, 43, 93, 152, 172, 174, 176-7, 180-1, 187-8
detoxify   140, 203-5
DHEA   106, 113-14, 116, 136, 138

E

EFT (emotional freedom technique)   9, 13, 54, 77, 117, 122, 169, 199, 274-6, 280
ego mind   27, 55, 73-4
emotions   22, 48, 52, 54-9, 61-2, 64-5, 68, 71, 74-8, 111, 121, 219, 277, 287, 295
energy   51-2, 55, 59-68, 71, 74, 76, 97, 105, 110-13, 115-16, 130, 262-3, 265, 271-3, 275
environment   45, 56, 68-9, 82-3, 125, 141, 178, 183, 200-1, 203, 208, 230, 257
estradiol   100, 130-2, 138
estriol   130-2, 138
estrogen   120, 125, 128-35, 137-41, 145, 154, 174, 204, 239, 247
estrogen dominance   134, 139
estrone   130-2, 134, 138

F

Fish Oil   155-8, 175
flu shot   216-18
flu vaccine   104, 210, 216-18

Made in the USA
Monee, IL
27 January 2022

89952762R00167